Basic Accounting for Hospital-Based Nonfinancial Managers

Basic Accounting for Hospital-Based Nonfinancial Managers

Sandra H. Pelfrey

Delmar Publishers Inc.®

NOTICE TO THE READER

Cover design by Anne Pompeo, Pompeo Designs

Delmar Staff:

Executive Editor: David Gordon
Project Editor: Carol Micheli
Production Coordinator: Bruce Sherwin
Design Coordinator: Karen Kemp

For information, address:
Delmar Publishers Inc.
2 Computer Drive, West, Box 15-015
Albany, NY   12212-9985

Copyright © 1992
BY DELMAR PUBLISHERS INC.

Printed in the United States of America
Published simultaneously in Canada
by Nelson Canada,
a division of The Thomson Corporation

10 9 8 7 6 5 4 3 2 1

Library of Congress Cataloging-in-Publication Data

Pelfrey, Sandra H.
    Basic accounting for hospital based nonfinancial managers/Sandra H. Pelfrey.
        p.   cm.
    Includes index.
    ISBN 0-8273-4894-0 — ISBN 0-8273-4895-9
    1. Hospitals — Accounting. I. Title.
    [DNLM: 1. Accounting. 2. Financial Management, Hospital. WX 157 P382b]
    HF5686.H7P38   1992
    657'.8322 — dc20
    DNLM/DLC
    for Library of Congress   91-28529
                                                                        CIP

Contents

Preface

This text is designed to give the nonfinancial health practitioner a general understanding of accounting and its processes, terminology, and end products, especially as they impact individual managers.

The accounting process generates reports that communicate operating information using a financial format. Accounting functions best when all readers of these reports understand the information being conveyed and can adapt their performance and that of their department in response to this information.

The text is divided into two sections. The first section presents an overview of the accounting process and financial statements and provides a general understanding of accounting terminology and its processes. It should help the reader develop a perspective of where and how individual departments relate to the entity.

The second section covers such operating and managerial topics as budgeting, both short- and long-term, cost identification, and behavior patterns. It also presents techniques for solving practical problems that individual managers encounter when preparing budgets and later evaluating actual performance.

The text is designed as a reference manual to give nonfinancial managers an understanding of accounting terminology, processes, and communication tools.

Introduction

Webster's International Dictionary defines accounting as the act of recounting or explaining. We have all been called upon at some time to give an accounting of what happened during a particular period of time. Accountants accomplish a similar task using general purpose financial statements which classify and summarize events that impact an entity using dollars and cents instead of text.

Accounting as a business function is defined as the art and science of recording, classifying, summarizing, and analyzing business transactions. This multiple part definition can be best understood by dividing it into its many parts. The basis of all accounting is the business transaction, which occurs when two parties meet and agree to an exchange. In general, the agreement itself does not constitute a transaction, even though a legal contract may have been signed. To be considered a business transaction, an agreement must be acted upon by exchanging goods or services.

Accountants use specific processes to record and summarize business transactions. The results of thousands of these transactions can be included within one set of financial statements, which is commonly referred to as the financial report.

The financial report consists of the following four individual statements. Each describes one aspect of the business by displaying specific, relevant information.

Financial Statements

1. **Balance Sheet.** Lists all of the resources owned and available to the institution at one point in time. It also lists the classes of individuals or companies that supply these resources.
2. **Income Statement.** Displays a summary of operating information that indicates whether the entity was able to cover its costs for a specific period of time.
3. **Statement of Equity.** Explains the change that has occurred in the owner's investment (termed equity) in the entity since the last financial report was issued.

4. **Cash Flow Statement.** Displays the inflows and outflows of cash throughout the period which result in the ending cash balance.

SUMMARY

Each financial statement provides readers with information regarding operations and current resources and their use during the period of time covered by the report.

SECTION *I*

Overview

I

History of Accounting

CHAPTER OBJECTIVES

1. Trace the evolution of the accounting function.
2. Look at the current environment of business.
3. Identify users of financial information.

Accounting in its very basic form can be traced back to the Middle Ages when explorers presented their sponsoring merchant a report of how they used the funds on their expeditions to the Orient. The current method of accounting, referred to as the double entry method, is based upon the premise that every business transaction involves an exchange in which something is given for something received. It can be traced to the fifteenth century writings of Friar Luca Pacioli and is estimated to have been in use for over 200 years prior to his documentation.

The business environment has changed greatly since those early times. There are many small and, oftentimes, family-operated businesses that exist today. However, large, often multinational, corporations provide the majority of goods and services sold in today's marketplace. These large corporate entities produce enormous volumes of goods and services and require great amounts of capital investment.

Technology has also played an important role in the development of large corporations. As a result of major technological advancements, the business world has evolved into a large complex society which often transcends geographical boundaries. Because of its rapid growth and complexity, business relies heavily upon the accounting function to gather and communicate financial information to owners, managers, and creditors.

As the business environment becomes complex, accountants continue to use the basic principles that have evolved over time as the basis for deciding how complex transactions should be recorded and reported. While the primary rules have not changed, they have been applied and interpreted to fit current situations.

USERS OF FINANCIAL INFORMATION _____

Management

To maintain control over a growing organization, management has to create an efficient, internal communication system. This system enables management to monitor daily operations and at the same time communicate with all units of an organization. To be efficient, a business needs free-flowing communication channels that contain a constant flow of timely, accurate information.

Communication is a two-way street. Information flows down from top management to all levels of the organization in the form of plans, budgets, operating goals, and directives. It flows upward as individual managers report their performance and adherence to the organization's goals and objectives. Performance reports take the form of periodic revenue and expense statements and are especially useful when compared to budgeted amounts. It is this feedback that enables management to determine whether goals can been achieved.

Managers at all levels need information that helps them identify potential problems as soon as possible. This is especially true as organizations expand and more departments and managerial levels are placed between the chief operating officer and employees who actually perform the daily operating functions.

Owners (Board of Trustees)

Owners need information about the soundness and profitability of the institution, especially in today's environment where the owner and manager can be and usually are different individuals. Small businesses may be able to operate with minimal written internal communication, financial or otherwise, because owners are intricately involved in all phases of daily operations. Some owners even have what can be termed a "sixth sense" and instinctively know how their business is performing and when and what to modify to improve operations.

Large corporations often have several thousand individual owners who are located throughout the world. In these instances, owners have an acute need for reliable financial data to enable them to evaluate the company's financial position, its progress, and management's ability to manage.

The Board of Trustees of a not-for-profit hospital accepts many of the responsibilities associated with business ownership. It is their duty to oversee operations and ensure that the hospital continues to operate and fulfill its stated purpose.

Creditors

Creditors are individuals or companies that loan money to an entity. Creditors use financial statements along with other data to assess a borrower's ability to repay loans on time.

Vendors

Vendors are special types of creditors who provide businesses with their required goods and services. These goods and services are provided in good faith with the expectation of receiving full payment at a later date. Financial statements and past credit histories furnish vendors information needed to support credit sales.

Employees

Employees are also vendors who agree to provide their labor on a regular basis in exchange for future wages. Employees must feel confident that their employer will continue operating, and thus continue paying their wages. Often employees, or their elected representatives, base their judgment of future ability to pay and the level of pay upon past performance. Financial statements furnish this information.

Government

Governmental units also require and utilize financial statement information. It may serve as the basis for taxing for-profit entities, or as a resource for formulating domestic policy or regulations for specific industries and/or certain transactions.

SUMMARY ———————————————————————

Accounting traces its beginnings to the Middle Ages. While its processes remain unchanged it has had to reinterpret fundamental principles in light of a changing economy. There is a continued need for financial information that communicates how well a business or organization is operating within its environment.

There are many users of financial information including management, owners or boards of trustees, creditors, vendors, employees, and governmental units. Each user poses different questions and has unique financial information needs. The accounting function is charged with furnishing relevant, reliable financial information in a form that is easily understood.

QUESTIONS ———————————————————————

1. Who are the various users of financial information? Discuss how their information needs may vary.
2. Which financial statement(s) would be of the most interest to
   1) management?
   2) boards of trustees?
   3) creditors?
   4) vendors?
   5) employees?
   6) government?

II

Environment of Accounting

CHAPTER OBJECTIVES

1. Explain basic accounting assumptions that have been made about the environment in which accounting must function.
2. Identify and explain the nature of generally accepted accounting principles.

The Industrial Revolution and the evolution of large corporations brought the need to communicate financial information to a broad range of interested parties. Over time, it has become necessary to standardize the basic accounting rules that form the foundation for the financial statements. Knowledge of these basic rules gives statement readers the ability to read and understand how an entity has performed in the economic environment. It also facilitates comparisons between companies in the same industry as well as between different times in the life of one company.

To aid in the process of formulating and communicating basic accounting rules or principles, accountants banded together and formed the professional organization known as the American Institute of Certified Public Accountants (AICPA). Established in 1887, the AICPA documents and communicates generally accepted accounting principles in use. Generally accepted accounting principles are defined as:

"the consensus at any time as to which economic resources and obligations should be recorded as assets and liabilities, which changes in them should be recorded, how the recorded assets and liabilities and changes in them should be measured, what information should be disclosed and how it should be disclosed, and which financial statements should be prepared." (AICPA, 1953)

Many of the basic accounting principles of 1887 remain unchanged today. Nonaccountants should have a cursory knowledge and understanding of generally accepted accounting principles in order to appreciate the information contained in financial statements.

ENVIRONMENT OF ACCOUNTING ─────────────

The financial report communicates company information such as what resources it owns, the debts it owes, its owners' investments, and how well it is performing operationally. The primary objective of the financial report is to furnish its readers with relevant, reliable financial information.

Generally accepted accounting principles (GAAP) allow for some flexibility between and among companies and industries. Because some variety exists, the specific accounting principles used by an entity must be disclosed within the financial report and then be used consistently. Before GAAP could be discerned, accountants had to agree on certain assumptions regarding the business environment and the role of accountants. The following assumptions serve as the foundation for GAAP.

Objectivity

The objectivity assumption states that accountants should act as independent recorders of business transactions. They must have verifiable, independently obtained information before a business transaction can be recorded. Public acceptance of the accounting function and financial reports depends on a belief in the integrity of the accounting profession and the credibility of the information related. Objectivity gives that needed credibility.

Entity

The entity assumption states that a business is separate and distinct from its owner(s). Financial records reflect the business transactions of the named entity only. Transactions affecting the owner(s) are recorded only to the extent that they also affect the business. Such transactions include the following:

1. additional investments made by owners, and
2. dividends or other withdrawals paid to the owners.

All other personal, owner-related receipts and payments are excluded from the financial records of the entity.

Going Concern

The going concern assumption states that, unless facts show otherwise, an entity is expected to continue operations. The entity exists now, and it is assumed that it will last indefinitely. Noted exceptions to the going concern assumption include organizations that are established for a limited time or activity, or those organizations that are unable to generate profits and are therefore unlikely to be able to continue operations. All other institutions are considered to have an ongoing existence.

Periodicity

The periodicity assumption states that even though the life of the entity is indefinite, it should be broken into uniform time periods for financial reporting purposes. The maximum time to be covered by a financial report is one year. Many large businesses have chosen to prepare monthly financial statements for internal use. Short time periods enable operating changes as well as changes in the economy to surface faster. Management can use this information to identify sporadic versus permanent economic trends and changes, and to determine what management action is needed.

Monthly financial reports are expensive because they require extra work. However, the added benefit of having current information generally outweighs their additional cost.

GENERALLY ACCEPTED ACCOUNTING PRINCIPLES

Using the previously mentioned assumptions, accountants further identified generally accepted accounting principles that dictate when a business transaction occurs, its classification, and the value to be recorded. The following principles or rules serve as the framework for the financial report.

Stable Dollar

The stable dollar principle specifies that all business transactions be recorded in terms of a common monetary unit, such as the U.S. dollar. For lack of an objectively determined alternative for valuation, the monetary unit is assumed to be stable. This concept assumes that today's dollar has the same intrinsic value as yesterday's or tomorrow's dollar. The effect of inflation is not readily apparent nor reflected in the financial report. Footnote disclosure may prove necessary to communicate this information.

Materiality

The principle of materiality states that financial statements must be correct in all important (material) aspects. It is impossible and impractical for financial data to be perfectly accurate. Accountants regularly use reasonable estimates to approximate revenues or expenses that are imprecise in nature. However, all important financial information should be included within the report.

Materiality is a relative amount and cannot be quantified for all entities. For example, $1,000 is an important or material amount to most individuals, but it would be considered unimportant or immaterial to many large corporations. In fact, most large corporations round all amounts in their financial statements to the nearest thousand dollar. Therefore, if an item is misstated by $1,000, it would not impair a reader's ability to assess a corporation's soundness or profitability.

Materiality, as defined by the law, is that amount that would cause a prudent person to change his/her mind about the reasonableness of financial information. Accountants apply the material principle by determining that all major financial data is fairly presented.

Consistency

There are instances when entities may choose between several general accounting principles. Practicality as well as cost-flow assumptions often dictate which principle is selected. In these situations, it is essential that the same principle be used from one financial report to the next. Therefore, the impact of a specific assumption is minimized and financial trends can be identified.

The consistency principle requires that financial data be prepared using the same cost- and/or revenue-flow assumptions as long as those assumptions prove reasonable. If an assumption is revised, readers must be alerted to 1) a change that has occurred, 2) the reasons for the change, and 3) the impact of the change on current and prior years' reported data. Therefore, readers can rely upon the consistent use of accounting principles throughout the reported period and from one period to the next.

Disclosure

The disclosure principle emphasizes the need to include all relevant financial information in the financial report. Many times, this cannot be accomplished within specific statements. It then becomes necessary to furnish additional information as footnotes to the statements. Footnotes and any other required disclosures are an integral part of any financial report and should be reviewed.

Cost

The cost principle states that historical cost is the only objective supportable value for recording resources. Cost is the amount paid to acquire an asset through an arms-length transaction in which both parties bargain with their own best interests in mind. As a result of this principle, an automobile would be valued at the final amount paid, not at the asking price that the dealer wanted or at the resale value that its current owner could receive if he or she were to sell the vehicle. As long as it is the owner's intention, its current selling price is undeterminable and meaningless. Historical cost governs the value at which assets are recorded.

Realization

An entity exists to provide services or goods to consumers. The realization principle states that revenue should be recorded when it is earned, and it is earned when an entity performs a service or sells a good regardless of whether payment is made.

Matching

To determine if an entity is operating profitably, it is necessary to compare all revenues generated for a given time period with all resources that were used up (expenses) to generate those revenues. The matching principle furnishes the rationale for deciding when an asset is exhausted becoming an expense. If the resource was used during the time period and/or directly to generate revenue, it should be expensed.

Conservatism

In addition to defining basic accounting assumptions and generally accepted accounting principles, accountants adopt a conservative view regarding gains and losses. This means that any and all losses are recorded as losses as soon as it is probable that they exist and that they can be estimated. As soon as a loss is probable, it must be recorded and disclosed to all interested parties even if it requires booking an estimation. Gains, however, are not recorded until all events giving rise to them transpire and they are a certainty.

SUMMARY

Accounting makes four assumptions about the nature of accounting information and its environment: 1) all recorded financial information must be objectively determined and supportable; 2) financial information for the accounting entity must be kept separated from that of the owner(s); 3) all accounting entities are assumed to be going concerns with indefinite lives unless information to the contrary is found; and 4) the indefinite lives of accounting entities must be divided into reporting time periods so that managers can provide relevant, financial information to all interested parties.

In addition to making basic assumptions about the accounting environment, the accounting profession has adopted fundamental rules called generally accepted accounting principles (GAAP). These principles dictate when transactions occur; what information must be recorded; and how that information will be valued, reported, and disclosed within financial statements.

REFERENCE

American Institute of Certified Public Accountants, Accounting Research Bulletin No. 43, (1953), Chap. 3A, par 11.

QUESTIONS

1. Why is it necessary to identify any assumptions that accountants have made concerning the business environment?
2. What are generally accepted accounting principles?
3. Explain how the matching principle and the realization principle reduce an entity's ability to manipulate numbers and create any net income desired?
4. The stable dollar principle has fallen under much criticism during periods of inflation. Discuss what alternatives might be used to value assets during periods of inflation. Comment on these.
5. Cost is the accounting principle that is used as the basis for recording assets. Why is the cost principle said to be the objective method of determining an asset's value?

EXERCISES

Matching

For each statement given below, select the item from the listing of terms that best identifies the principle or convention explained.

A. Conservatism
B. Consistency
C. Cost
D. Entity
E. Going Concern
F. Matching
G. Materiality

    H. Realization

    I.   Stable Dollar

___ 1. The accountant will record a loss if it is probable that one exists, but will wait to record a gain until it is a certainty.

___ 2. No attempt is made to update the value of a building that was purchased in 1967 for $100,000, but has an appraised value of $300,000.

___ 3. It is assumed that the organization will exist tomorrow; therefore, a resource can be established as an asset when it is purchased even though it is intended to be used up at a later time.

___ 4. One dollar paid is assumed to have purchasing power equal to that of another dollar that is paid at another time.

___ 5. The institution borrowed money from the bank. Repayment with interest is due at the end of one year, which is two months from now. Interest is recorded as owed at the end of this month so that financial statements can be prepared.

___ 6. Revenue is recorded as earned when services are provided even though it is uncertain whether the consumer will be able to pay for the services.

___ 7. A hospital also operates a nursing school and is very careful to keep revenue and expenses for its nursing school separate from those of the hospital.

___ 8. Patients come and go throughout the day. The hospital uses the patient census that is taken at midnight as a basis for charging patients for a hospital room.

___ 9. The accounting system expenses all equipment that costs less than $100, even though it satisfies the definition of fixed assets.

III

General Purpose Financial Statements

CHAPTER OBJECTIVES

1. Discuss the nature of financial statements.
   A. Balance Sheet
   B. Income Statement
   C. Statement of Equity
   D. Cash Flow Statement
2. Explain the components of each statement.
3. Explain relationships that exist among and between the financial statements.
4. Discuss the various forms of ownership that exist, the advantages and disadvantages of each, and how that ownership affects financial statements.

As discussed previously, the accountant's role is one of communicator and the accountant's tools are the four financial statements. These financial statements include:

1. The Balance Sheet
2. The Income Statement
3. The Statement of Owners' Equity
4. The Cash Flow Statement

It is necessary to view the interrelationship of all four financial statements to fully understand an organization's financial position and operations. While one statement furnishes useful information, it is incomplete.

The statements and their contents are explained in this chapter. The examples given are for-profit businesses whose owners are rewarded with profit distributions. A primary purpose of for-profit companies is to generate profits that are distributed to owners in the form of dividends or withdrawals. Differences exist between for-profit and not-for-profit entities, as well as between different forms of for-profit organizations. These differences exist in fact and are reflected within the owners' equity section of the balance sheet. The various forms of ownership are discussed later in this chapter.

BALANCE SHEET

The balance sheet (sometimes referred to as the statement of financial position) lists the resources (assets) that an organization has at its disposal at one point in time. By definition, an asset is any resource that has future value beyond the date of the listing. Like individuals, business entities possess many and varied assets. Some common assets include cash, investments, property, buildings, furnishings, and automobiles. All of these items have one thing in common. They are resources that have value, exist now, and are expected to be of value or available for use tomorrow.

The balance sheet also identifies the two general groups of investors who are responsible for providing an entity's assets — creditors and owners. Resources borrowed from creditors or purchased with the promise of future payment are referred to as liabilities. Liabilities are debts that carry specific repayment amounts that may or may not require interest in addition to the original amount borrowed.

The second source of assets is the organization's owners. This is commonly referred to as owners' equity. Owners' equity includes the original investment that owners made at the start of the business plus any excess of income over expenses derived from operations that remains undistributed to owners. Unlike creditors who have loaned the business a specific amount expecting exact repayment, owners invest in a business with the expectation of increasing their initial investment with funds that the company generates. Owners are never guaranteed a profit. In fact, they often suffer losses as a result of operations and losses that effectively reduce the value of owners' equity. Profit or loss uncertainty is a risk inherent to owners.

A company does not have to distribute all of its profits to its owners. Management often accumulates profits and uses them as a basis for financing expansion and new projects or product lines. That which is not reinvested in the company may be distributed to owners in the form of dividends. Reinvested earnings increase owners' equity; dividends or withdrawals decrease it.

Since every resource must come from somewhere, the balance sheet is supported by the following formula.

$$\text{Assets} = \text{Liabilities} + \text{Owners Equity}$$

This means that resources are equal to the amounts invested by creditors and owners. Both sides of the equation must equal or be in balance.

Assets

The balance sheet lists all assets the entity possesses. The assets could be combined into one total for statement presentation and be listed, for example, as: Total Assets, $10,000. Balance sheet readers generally find the detail composition of these assets important. The user of financial data would have different perceptions of similar entities whose total assets each totalled $10,000 if one company's asset is cash and the second one's is $10,000 of real estate. From the user's perspective, it is important to know the kinds and amounts of individual assets that an entity owns. Accountants therefore keep separate accounts for different business assets.

To make a balance sheet more meaningful and easier to read, assets are separated into two major categories. The first category is referred to as current assets or resources with future values that are expected to be converted into cash or used up within the next year. Examples of current assets include cash, inventories, supplies, and accounts receivable.

Long-term assets form the second category of assets. These are resources whose useful life is expected to extend beyond one year. Examples of long-term assets include land, buildings, equipment, and automobiles. All of these long-term assets are examples of fixed assets or property, plant, and equipment. The long-term category may be further divided as needed. For example, an entity may own investments in negotiable stocks or corporate debt securities. If this is the case, it is best to separate these long-term investments from property, plant, and equipment because the total of the two asset groups is meaningless and confusing. Separating these items into separate categories such as fixed assets and investment facilitates better understanding.

Current Assets   The most commonly used current asset accounts are listed and described below.

Cash — Money that an organization has on hand or in a checking or savings account that is readily available for disbursement as needed.

Marketable Securities — Negotiable securities that can be easily transferred or will mature within one year. These securities may include government securities, corporate or municipal debt securities, and common stock. The intention of the entity dictates whether these are classified as current or long-term. If the entity intends selling its securities if cash is needed, the securities are classified as current assets.

Accounts Receivable — Accounts receivable represents the entity's legal right to receive money at a future date for unpaid goods and services that have been provided to a customer or patient.

Note Receivable — The legal right to receive money from another entity evidenced by a signed promissory note. If the note falls due within the next year, the note is classified as a current asset. If repayment is not required within the next year, the note receivable is considered long-term.

Inventory — Merchandise or goods that were purchased with the intention of reselling them to future consumers, and not for use by the entity.

Prepaid Expenses — Items that have been paid for in advance that will be used in future time periods. Supplies are resources that are expected to be used during operations. These are listed as prepaid expenses until they are in fact used. Other prepaid items include insurance premiums and prepaid rent.

Long-term Assets   Long-term assets are those assets that are considered to have a life of greater than one year. Listed below are some examples of long-term assets. Next to each asset is a brief description of the contents of that account.

Fixed Assets or Property, Plant, and Equipment — The cost of real assets such as buildings, machinery, furnishings, and automobiles.

Each of these assets has a useful life of more than one year. In addition, these assets must physically exist and be used in daily operations.

Investments — Assets that are purchased as a source of revenue or for use at a later time. These assets include real estate, corporate stocks, and bonds that an entity intends to keep for more than one year.

Liabilities

Liabilities are amounts owed to various creditors and are classified by their nature and to whom the debt is owed. As with assets, liabilities are divided into two categories: current and long-term. Current liabilities are those debts that are expected to be repaid within one year's time, resulting in a transfer of current assets. Long-term liabilities are those debts that are expected to be repaid after the twelve-month period.

Current Liabilities   Some examples of current liabilities follow. A brief explanation of each is also given.

Accounts Payable — Amounts owed to vendors who supply goods or services that are purchased to meet operational needs, such as utilities, food, pharmaceuticals, linens, and dressings. These items have been delivered, but their corresponding invoices remain unpaid at the time financial statements are prepared.

Notes Payable — Monies that are borrowed, generally from financial institutions, and for which an entity has signed a legal promissory note that specifies when the money will be repaid. If repayment is to be within the next twelve months, it is considered a current liability. If the note is to be repaid more than one year from the balance sheet date, it is considered a long-term liability.

Salaries Payable — Amounts owed to employees for hours they have worked but for which they have not yet been paid.

Payroll Withholdings and Payroll Taxes — Amounts that an entity is required by law to deduct from employees' pay and must remit to various taxing bodies. Businesses must also pay taxes to various governmental units for the right to have employees. For example, an entity must match its employees' deductions for Social Security taxes, and must pay state and federal unemployment taxes.

Taxes Payable — Amounts that an entity owes various governmental units for taxes that are incurred as part of daily operations. These taxes may include sales, property, and income taxes.

Unearned Income or Deferred Income — Monies received from patients or customers as deposits against future services. Because these funds have not yet been earned, an entity is legally required to provide a service or refund these deposits, giving rise to a liability.

Long-term Liabilities Long-term or noncurrent liabilities are those legal obligations or debts that are owed and expected to be paid after one year from the balance sheet date.

Mortgage Payable — The amount that is legally owed as the result of purchasing real estate with borrowed funds. A mortgage is a legal document that states that the real estate is collateral for the loan. This permits the lender to sell the property for the balance of the debt owed should the borrower be unable to make the required payments.

Bonds Payable — There are times when an entity needs to borrow such large sums of money that one financial institution is unable to lend the entire amount. Bond markets are established for this purpose. Bonds are special promissory notes that carry promises to pay a specified dollar amount (principal) at some future or maturity date plus a specified rate of interest on the bond principal every six months. The interest rate, amount to be repaid, and date of repayment are all stated on the face of the bond. Most bonds mature (come due for repayment) within 20 to 40 years from their date of issue.

Other Long-term Debt — An entity may enter into legal arrangements other than those previously mentioned. Those debts and any relevant information pertaining to them must be disclosed in the balance sheet and its footnotes.

Owners' Equity

This section of the balance sheet displays the accumulated value related to the owners' investments plus any reinvested operating earnings. After reviewing the contents of the income statement, a reader will realize that the owners' equity section of a balance sheet connects these two financial statements. A separate financial statement entitled the Statement of Owners' Equity is prepared to reinforce the concept that income from operations (from the income statement) is the element that causes the change in owners' equity from one time period to the next. While the Statement of Owners' Equity explains the changes that occurred in the equity account during the period, the final balance is displayed in the balance sheet and becomes the amount that explains the owners' equity in the listed resources.

OPERATING or INCOME STATEMENT _____

An entity is in business or operates by providing services or selling goods. Because it is essential to know whether operations are profitable, and because an entity needs a positive equity balance to remain in existence, it is necessary to monitor and report the results of operations. An income statement accumulates and reports detailed relevant operating data under broad categories called revenue and expense.

Revenue is an active term and communicates total charges for work performed and earned during the period. Expenses are resources that an entity uses during the period in the process of generating revenue.

The formula that supports the income statement is:

$$Revenue - Expenses = Net \ Income \ or \ Loss$$

If total revenue is greater than total expenses:

$$Revenue - Expenses = Net \ Income$$

If total revenue is less than total expenses:

$$Revenue - Expenses = Net \ Loss$$

An Example of Revenue and Expense

On Saturday night, emergency room personnel acting as representatives of a hospital clean, stitch, and dress a patient's wound. The emergency room has provided a service for which the hospital is entitled to charge that patient; therefore, the emergency room has generated or earned revenue. This earning process occurred regardless of whether the patient pays at time of service, at a later date, or not at all.

Consequently, when payment is received at a later date, the hospital is merely exchanging assets, giving up the asset accounts receivable in exchange for cash.

In this example, emergency room personnel used supplies and staff time to treat the patient. Blood work, laboratory tests, and pharmaceuticals were ordered for the patient. Charges appeared on the patient's bill for these services. The cost of resources used to provide the services must be matched against the revenue and recorded as period expenses. Items such as salary, supplies, and other expenses must be included on the income statement. Analysis of these two factors (revenue and expense) determines whether operations are profitable.

Categories of Revenue and Expense

Various revenue categories are industry-specific and are established for comparison reasons. The most common operating revenue categories used by health care providers are:

1. Inpatient nursing service revenue
2. Inpatient ancillary service revenue
3. Outpatient revenue

Secondary sources of revenue such as cafeteria sales, investment income, and contributions also exist.

Operating expenses are generally displayed using one of two classification methods. The first method lists expenses by type including, but not limited to, the following:

1. Salaries and employee benefits
2. Supplies
3. Expenses
4. Depreciation
5. Interest
6. Insurance

Expenses can also be classified by function. The most commonly reported functions are listed below.

1. Nursing service
2. Ancillary departments
3. Physical plant

4. General administration
5. Depreciation
6. Interest
7. Insurance

Regardless of expense reporting classification, its consistent use will furnish information necessary for understanding operations and making intelligent decisions regarding operations.

STATEMENT OF OWNERS' EQUITY _____

The owners' equity account is the means of connecting two balance sheets using the results of operations that were reported in the income statement. Because of the importance of this information, businesses prepare a separate financial statement, the Statement of Owners' Equity, to disclose the changes that have occurred in the equity account since the last financial report was issued. The statement will reconcile the amount that was last reported on the balance sheet to the amount that is currently being reported as the balance of owners' equity. (Detailed information included in the statement will depend upon the form of ownership that the organization has chosen.)

FORMS OF OWNERSHIP _____

There are different legal forms under which companies can be organized. It is important to note that regardless of ownership, all other business transactions are recorded exactly the same. The name of an entity will not always disclose its form of ownership. The only way to be certain of its form is to look at the owners' equity statement. The three forms of ownership are:

1. Sole proprietorship
2. Partnership
3. Corporation

Sole Proprietorship

A sole proprietorship is a business entity that has only one owner. That individual accepts all risks associated with operations and is entitled to

R.J. Jones balance, January 1, 1992	$10,000
Add income earned for the year	6,000
Subtotal	16,000
Less withdrawals made by owner in 1992	5,000
R.J. Jones balance, December 31, 1992	$11,000

Figure 3.1. Statement of Owner's Equity for a sole proprietor.

all of its profits and losses. A sole proprietor invests assets and forms a new entity. There is unlimited legal liability associated with sole proprietorships because under the law, a sole proprietor and his/her business are viewed as one entity. Any business debts may be satisfied with the owner's private assets and, conversely, business assets may be used to satisfy the owner's personal debts.

In addition to unlimited liability, the sole proprietorship has a limited legal lifetime. Its life coincides with that of its owner. If an owner decides to stop operating a sole proprietorship, the easiest way to accomplish this is simply to close up shop. A sole proprietorship ends when additional owners are added or when the entire business is sold to someone else. Because of its ease in establishing and ceasing operations, sole proprietorships are considered the easiest form of ownership.

Because of its unlimited liability and limited life, the sole proprietor's total assets are effectively limited to those invested by or able to be borrowed by one person. For this reason, sole proprietorships are generally relatively small in size.

The statement of owner's equity gives a summary of its owner's account for the current year. The net income, shown as an addition to equity, can be traced directly to reported net income on the income statement.

An example of the statement of owner's equity for a sole proprietor is depicted in Figure 3.1. From the information depicted in Figure 3.1, readers can gather that there is only one owner, that the owner's name is R.J. Jones, and that his/her investment in the business entity amounts to $11,000.

Partnership

Businesses can also be organized as partnerships, where two or more owners have agreed to establish and operate it under a general partner-

R.J. Jones balance, December 31, 1992	$12,000
S.T. Smith balance, December 31, 1992	9,500
L.K. Meyers balance, December 31, 1992	7,400
Total partnership equity	$28,900

Figure 3.2. Owners' equity section of the balance sheet for a partnership.

ship agreement. For accounting purposes, the business entity is separate from its owners; however, the law again views a partnership and its owners as one. Partnerships, like sole proprietorships, have unlimited liability.

Also, as with sole proprietorships, a partnership has a lifetime limited to that of any one of its partners. It will cease to exist when any partner leaves or when a new partner is admitted to the business.

Partners invest in an entity; they share profits in a ratio that is agreed upon; and each is entitled to withdraw his/her investment once creditors have been satisfied. Because a partnership requires input from more than one person, its total accumulated assets are greater than those of just one individual.

As in the case of a sole proprietorship, the remainder of the balance sheet remains unchanged. It would be impossible to detect an entity's form of ownership by reading asset and liability detail. It is only by examining its statement of owners' equity and the equity section of its balance sheet that the form of ownership can be discovered.

An example of the owners' equity section of the balance sheet for a partnership appears in Figure 3.2. There would be separate statements of owners' equity for each of the partners that would provide detailed analysis of the division of profits or losses, as well as the amount of each partner's asset withdrawals.

Corporation

Both accounting and the law agree on the entity recognition of corporations. Individuals invest in corporations when they purchase shares of stock which serve as evidence of ownership. Each share's owner has a limited liability, meaning that the maximum loss an individual can sustain is the amount that was paid for the initial investment.

Because they are separate legal entities, corporations have indefinite lives that are not in any way linked to the lives of its other owners.

Their ability to sell shares and exist indefinitely helps corporations amass large amounts of assets. For this reason, major United States industries are organized as corporations.

There may be several different classes of stock within one corporation, with the common shareholder being the most basic shareholder. If more than one class of stock is issued, the owners' equity section of a corporation's balance sheet is required by law to keep amounts paid for each class of stock in separate accounts. Any profits or retained earnings that have been generated by operations and remain undistributed are carried in a separate account called retained earnings.

An example of the owners' or shareholders' equity section of the balance sheet of a corporation is shown in Figure 3.3. Details of changes within equity accounts are reported in a separate statement of stockholders' equity.

Not-for-profit entities generally select the corporate form of organization because of its indefinite legal life. This enables an entity to amass large amounts of resources or assets, because creditors know that it will have an indefinite life.

Most not-for-profit health care corporations originated through donations. Original donors or investors may have been religious orders, governmental units, or communities. The founding fathers of these not-for-profit entities promised that any earnings generated by the entity would be retained and reinvested in the entity. No outside owners receive profit or dividend distributions.

The existence of not-for-profit corporations does not create a need for new financial statements. The only change in presentation occurs within the equity section of its balance sheet and statement of owners' equity (referred to as fund or net asset balance).

It is essential that a not-for-profit organization record its equity because creditors and suppliers require this information. It may also be required by employee groups, contributors, and governmental units. An example of the statement of owners' equity can be found in Figure 3.4.

Common Stock, 100,000 shares	$100,000
Retained Earnings	22,000
Total Shareholders' Equity	$122,000

Figure 3.3. Owners' or shareholders' equity section of the balance sheet of a corporation.

Beginning Balance	$125,000
Add net income for the year	10,000
Balance, end of year	$135,000

Figure 3.4. Statement of Owners' Equity for a not-for-profit organization.

A not-for-profit organization appoints respected members of the community to serve as members of its board of trustees. These trustees have a legal responsibility to be knowledgeable about the entity's operating activity. Collectively, they determine its direction, and are empowered to borrow monies in its name and to hire a management team.

CASH FLOW STATEMENT

Because revenue is not directly related to cash receipts nor expenses to cash disbursements, it is possible for an institution to report sizeable net income and suffer a shortage of cash. Reasons for changes in cash may not be apparent to an untrained reader and may even lead readers to doubt an entity's reporting credibility. The fourth required financial statement, the cash flow statement, was created to fill this void and furnish information needed to evaluate management's ability to effectively use its cash resource.

Management's responsibilities include operating profitably and financing operations in such a manner that an entity accepts that level of debt that can be repaid without risking its collapse or takeover. Prior to the cash flow statement, detailed financing and investment information were buried in the financial report. The cash flow statement assembles all of this information in one place.

Cash Generated by Operations
+ (-) Cash from Investment Decisions
+ (-) Cash from Financial Decisions
Net Change in the Cash Account

Figure 3.5. Formula for the cash flow statement.

The formula supporting the cash flow statement appears in Figure 3.5. The cash flow statement is divided into three sections. The first section recreates a cash operating statement; the second section summarizes investment decisions (namely the purchases and sales of long-term assets); and the final section of this statement discloses those financing decisions that management made during the year. Financing decisions relate to the acquisition and repayment of long-term debt and owners' equity transactions.

Cash generated by operations combined with cash generated or used for investment transactions plus cash generated or used for financing transactions explains the change in the cash account over the period. This statement explains how an entity can be profitable and have less cash at the end of the year than it had at the beginning.

Frequency of Financial Statement Preparation

The periodicity principle recognizes that even though an entity has an indefinite life, it is still necessary to report on operations at regular intervals of time. This gives financial statement users interim information concerning an entity's profitability and solvency. An entity must prepare annual financial statements. The Internal Revenue Code requires annual tax returns from individuals and businesses alike, and from not-for-profit as well as from for-profit corporations. More importantly, good management principles dictate that managers be informed on a regular basis of an entity's financial progress.

A small organization commonly breaks its lifetime into periods of a year because management is closer to operations in smaller organizations, and the use of a year as the basis of formal financial statements may be satisfactory for statement users. Owners and managers can monitor one or two accounts such as cash, accounts receivable, or sales and gather necessary operating information.

A larger organization is much more complex in structure and requires more structured financial reports at regular intervals. These larger entities generally prepare monthly financial statements and accumulate year-to-date information at the same time.

One factor to be considered in preparing financial statements more frequently than once a year is the cost. Any additional benefits derived from having current information provided must be worth the additional cost of preparation. Sample financial statements are provided in Figure 3.6.

ASSETS		19__
UNRESTRICTED FUNDS		
CURRENT ASSETS		
Cash and short-term investments		$ 1,938,838
Accounts receivable:		
Patients, less allowances of		
$2,149,278 in 19__		9,286,670
Medicare		1,063,529
Other		73,134
Inventories		604,553
Prepaid expenses		523,297
TOTAL CURRENT ASSETS		13,490,021
BOARD-DESIGNATED		
Cash and short-term investments		2,785,932
Pooled investments—Note B		3,803,349
		6,589,281
ASSETS		
RESTRICTED TO USE		
Cash		39,697
Student Loans Receivable		297,866
Pooled Investments—Note B		1,900,850
Equity investments (approximate market $990,827)		794,240
Other Investments (approximate market $)		1,686,940
Real Estate		160,000
		4,879,593
SELF-INSURANCE TRUST—Note C		
Cash	48	
Investments (approximate market		
19__ —$1,719,564)	1,797,750	
		1,797,798
PROPERTY, PLANT, AND EQUIPMENT,		
less allowances for depreciation and		
amortization—Notes D, E, and H		28,029,202
		$54,785,895

Figure 3.6. Sample financial statements.

19__

LIABILITIES AND FUND BALANCES

UNRESTRICTED FUNDS	
CURRENT LIABILITIES	
Accounts payable	$ 2,255,410
Medicaid payable	248,951
Accrued salaries, wages, and payroll taxes	3,451,271
Accrued expenses	330,101
Deferred income	187,754
Current portion of long-term debt—Note E	433,198
Current portion of capital lease	
obligation—Note H	550,476
TOTAL CURRENT LIABILITIES	$ 7,457,161
LONG-TERM DEBT, less current portion—Note E	2,943,813
Note Payable to U.S. Government—Note F	124,600
CAPITAL LEASE OBLIGATION, less current	
portion—Note H	2,012,063
RESERVE FOR SELF-INSURANCE—Note C	1,797,798
OTHER NONCURRENT LIABILITIES	762,737
TOTAL LIABILITIES	15,098,172
FUND BALANCE	
Specific Purpose	2,010,156
Endowment	2,798,579
Unrestricted	34,878,988
TOTAL FUND BALANCE	39,687,723
	$54,785,895

Figure 3-6 (continued).

SUMMARY

There are four financial statements that together form the financial report. These four statements include: 1) the balance sheet that lists the resources and equity, both creditor and owner, of the entity; 2) the

SAMPLE HOSPITAL
STATEMENT OF REVENUES AND EXPENSES

19___

Net Patient Service Revenue	$62,274,039
Other Operating Revenue	2,455,194
Total Operating Revenue	64,729,233
Operating Expenses:	
Nursing Service	12,225,951
Ancillary Services	20,221,520
Building Services	5,946,401
Dietary Services	3,382,655
Administrative Services	6,129,081
Nursing and Medical Education	2,417,550
Employee Benefits	5,055,837
Bad Debt Expenses	2,207,537
Insurance	1,387,934
Depreciation	2,489,620
Interest	457,670
Other	626,623
	$62,548,379
Excess of Operating Revenues over Expenses	2,180,854
Nonoperating Revenue	
Contributions	293,467
Income from investments	1,106,566
	1,400,033
Excess of Revenues over Expenses	$3,580,887

Figure 3-6 (continued).

income statement that summarizes operations for the entity, displaying its major sources of revenue and expense; 3) the statement of owners' equity that analyzes the change in the owner's equity account from one period to the next; and 4) the cash flow statement that explains the change in the cash account for the period, identifying sources and uses of cash by the major activities of the entity. These four statements provide information that readers need to evaluate a specific entity and compare it to others in its industry.

SAMPLE HOSPITAL
CASH FLOW STATEMENT
For year ended December 31, 19___

Cash received from patient services		$58,261,406
Other Operating Revenues		2,416,760
		$60,678,166
Cash paid for Operating Expenses		(56,271,247)
Cash Inflow from Operations		4,406,919
Cash Contributions and Investment Income		1,400,039
		5,806,958
Investing		
Board Designated	(1,443,978)	
Self-insurance Trust Investment	(1,031,318)	
Purchase of Equipment	(3,888,245)	
Increase in Restricted Investment	(546,063)	(6,909,604)
Financing		
Paid L-T debt	(427,061)	
Increase noncurrent liabilities	399,556	
Paid Lease Principal	(390,172)	(417,677)
Reclassification		
Restricted gifts received	123,850	
Restricted income	309,453	
Reclassified to operations	(161,546)	
Grants to students	(5,131)	266,626
Decrease in Cash		($1,253,697)

Figure 3-6 (continued).

Forms of ownership include: 1) sole proprietorship (one owner), 2) partnerships (two or more owners), and 3) corporations. Most hospitals are organized as not-for-profit corporations with the only distinction from their for-profit counterparts being that not-for-profit entities do not distribute their profits outside the entity.

QUESTIONS _____

1. What four financial statements compose the financial report?
2. Give the formula that supports the balance sheet. What information is contained within this statement?

3. Give the formula that supports the income statement. What information is contained within this statement?
4. Give the formula that supports the statement of changes in equity. What information is contained within this statement?
5. Give the formula that supports the cash flow statement. What information is contained within this statement?
6. What ownership forms may an entity take? Give the advantages and disadvantages of each form.
7. Why is the corporate form preferred by most of the large companies?
8. Distinguish between not-for-profit and for-profit corporations.
9. Is it illegal or immoral for a not-for-profit entity to operate at a profit? Explain your answer.
10. What would be the result of a not-for-profit entity continually operating at a loss or just breaking even?

EXERCISES

Instructions

Sort out the accounts listed below. Identify them by their category of either asset, liability, equity, revenue, or expense. Then prepare the Balance Sheet, Income Statement, and Statement of Equity using these accounts.

Accounts Payable	$ 800
Accounts Receivable	$ 1,200
Bonds Payable	$10,000
Building	$15,000
Cash	$ 400
Equipment	$ 7,000
Equity (Fund Balance at beginning of the year)	$12,000
Expenses for the year	$17,300
Investments	$ 1,000
Inventory	$ 600
Land	$ 800
Revenue for the year	$20,000
Salaries Payable	$ 500

IV

The Accounting Cycle

1. Review the chain of events that leads to preparation of the financial report.
2. Explain the method of accumulating different types of business transactions.
3. Explain the need for accounting adjustment at the end of the accounting period.
4. Identify business transactions that are unique to the health care industry.

The accounting cycle is the time and chain of events needed to create a complete set of financial statements or a financial report. There are certain tasks that need to be done daily, weekly, biweekly, and monthly to accumulate necessary financial information. The time schedule assigned to each task will, in large measure, depend upon the volume of transactions to be recorded and the need to be able to review detailed data at various intervals between statement dates.

DAILY TRANSACTIONS

Patient Charges (Revenue)

Revenue from patient charges is recorded daily. Charge slips are produced by ordering services from pharmacy, laboratory, respiratory therapy, and other ancillary departments and serve as source documents for posting charges to patient accounts. They also give supplying departments credit for revenue generated.

Very few institutions hand-process charge slips, although some small institutions may have only slightly automated record keeping systems. Most institutions use computerized systems to record daily transactions fast and accurately. If charge slips are sent to data processing for inputting after services are rendered, the system is referred to as an off-line system. The computer stores all of one day's charges and updates patients' accounts during the late evening hours when hospital activities are reduced.

Some institutions use computer terminals instead of charge slips to order tests and medications and charge patient accounts. This type of system is referred to as an on-line system. On-line systems can update records at a later time; however, they generally update at the same time that the order is filled, making them an on-line, real-time system.

Benefits of on-line systems are great. They omit the need to prepare, transmit, and input paper charge slips, thus saving time and labor. On the other hand, the cost of an on-line system is extremely high because every ordering and operating department must have access to computer terminals that are connected with other departments of the institution and to a mainframe that accumulates all patient data.

Regardless of the computer system in use, patients' accounts must be updated regularly. A by-product of billing patients is the generation of revenue and activity data for all revenue-producing departments.

Cash Receipts

Cash receipts from patients, third-party payers, and other sources are also recorded daily. The cash receipt may come from direct patient payments and third-party insurance carriers and must be applied to the correct patient account as expeditiously as possible. Patient billing systems create new statements at regular intervals and it is essential that an institution maintain its credibility by timely posting of payments.

Credit Purchases of Supplies and Services

Another transaction that should be recorded frequently is credit purchases of supplies and services (other than employee services). This process, in itself, takes time because supplies and services are generally received at various locations throughout the hospital by individual departments or by a designated receiving department. Paperwork regarding actual receipt must be prepared and transmitted to an accounting department. After receiving report, invoice, and purchase order have been matched, verified, and approved, accounting records a liability and a purchase.

Cash Payments

After processing purchases, accounting prepares a request for payment. Whether or not a check is prepared immediately will depend upon whether all supporting paperwork is in order, whether the vendor requires payment at that time, and whether there is enough cash in the bank to cover the check. If it is decided to delay payment, the bill remains part of the liability balance. When payment is approved, the check is prepared, signed, and mailed, and the liability is removed.

TRANSACTIONS THAT ARE RECORDED WEEKLY

Payroll

The payroll function accumulates hours worked by employees and, using pay rates, converts them into payroll checks that adhere to federal, state, and local tax withholding requirements. Most institutions establish a separate department within accounting that tabulates hours, calculates gross pay and tax withholding, and issues and distributes payroll checks.

There are many ways to tabulate and summarize hours worked. Some institutions use time clocks that are placed at strategic internal locations. Using time cards, employees mark the start and end of each shift, letting the time clock record exact times. Some institutions may even require employees to clock in and out for lunch. If this practice is omitted, employees are presumed to have taken the allotted time for meals. Some institutions replace time cards with payroll time sheets. The employee's home department is responsible for maintaining and corroborating the number of hours worked. This job may fall to clerical staff or may be assigned to the departmental supervisor. Still other hospitals maintain sophisticated computer systems that keep track of each employee's hours and the department worked in. Whichever system is used to tabulate employee hours and pay, data must be processed weekly and stored until payroll checks are prepared and distributed.

Central Stores or Supplies

Another transaction that may be summarized and recorded weekly is the usage of central stores items. Some central stores items are billable items and can be charged directly to patients, while other items are nonchargeable supplies. These nonchargeable items are expensed directly to the using departments when they are issued. Departments with supply closets generally establish specific inventory levels and charge the using department when the supply closet is replenished. Some hospitals replenish department inventory supply closets daily; others may replenish them at less frequent intervals.

AT MONTH'S END ———————————————

Adjustments

When it is time to prepare financial statements, the realization and matching principles have to be reviewed against the accounts of the entity to ascertain that the income statement will reflect all major classes of revenue earned and all material expenses incurred for the time period. Since patient revenue is recorded daily, there is generally no need to enter any adjustment to accumulated amounts. No adjustments are required for expenses that properly reflect resources used during the period.

Five types of transactions require adjustment at period end to ensure that all revenue earned and expenses incurred have been recorded. Adjustments are needed for:

1. Revenues that are earned but not yet recorded
2. Monies that were initially recorded as unearned income or liabilities for which services have been provided, and the revenue earned
3. Resources that have been used up (expenses) before they have been recorded as a purchase

4. Resources that were recorded as assets when they were purchased and have subsequently been used up and need to be recorded as expenses
5. Depreciation

Revenues Earned But Not Recorded Because of methods used to record patient charges, the majority in an institution are recorded as they are earned. If an institution has any other revenue that has been earned but has not yet been recorded, an adjustment is required to record that income. Examples of earned but unrecorded revenue requiring adjustment are investment and interest income.

Deposits Some institutions require preadmission deposits from patients as a sign of good faith that are used to offset any patient charges. Deposits are liabilities when received because the institution owes the patient a refund or future service. Later, when the patient is admitted and charges are accumulated, the liability no longer exists. Accountants must physically adjust liability accounts to remove deposits that have been earned, transferring them to revenue accounts.

Expenses Incurred But Not Recorded Accounting will handle recording expenses when it processes invoices. Occasionally, some operating expenses need to be included in the current period before invoices are received. In these instances it may be necessary to estimate certain expenses to properly satisfy the matching principle. Adjustments are needed to include these expenses in the financial statements.

In general, month-end adjustments are needed for earned but unpaid payroll expenses. Monthly or bimonthly paid employees have no lag time between when they earn their wages and when they are paid. For them, salary expense is properly recorded in the month it is incurred. Most institutions pay on a weekly or biweekly basis, leaving employees with some hours that have been worked but unpaid at month's end. These unpaid work hours or days must be recorded as an expense and a liability for the period. Departmental records are adjusted for the increase in salary expense created by the adjustment.

An example of an accrued payroll adjustment appears in Figure 4.1. An analysis similar to this one will be made for every department within the institution.

Total salaries for a two-week period	$140,000
Number of days in the pay period	14
Average salary expense for one day	$ 10,000
Number of workdays that remain unpaid at the end of the month	4
Salary expense and liability adjustment at month's end	$ 40,000

Figure 4.1. An accrued payroll adjustment.

Assets That Have Become Expenses Over Time   Inventory items are assets when purchased and become expenses as they are used. The central stores system for charging nonchargeable supplies makes the required adjustment. Other asset-to-expense adjustments may be needed for such items as prepaid insurance related to property, liability, and malpractice policies. When premiums are paid, they are considered an asset because they give the institution the right to insurance coverage for future time periods, or the right to a refund if the policy is canceled before its renewal date. Each month an entry must be made to record another month's expense and reduce the asset by the amount that has been used.

Depreciation   Depreciation is allocation of the cost of a fixed asset (building, machinery, equipment, and furnishings) to the time periods that it serves. Estimates of the asset's life and salvage value are two of the items used in calculating depreciation charges for the time period. The difference between a fixed asset's cost and salvage value is the amount that the institution will use up or expense over that asset's life.

The straight-line method of depreciating fixed assets is the simplest depreciation method. There are other, more complex methods that will not be discussed in this text. All serve the same function of systematically charging the cost of fixed assets to the periods they serve. An example of a straight-line depreciation calculation of a fixed asset can be found in Figure 4.2.

Accountants prepare depreciation adjustments for all fixed assets owned. With the advent of computers, the magnitude of this task has been greatly reduced. Computers are able to rapidly calculate and record periodic depreciation for all fixed assets that are used in operations.

Fixed asset information:	
Asset cost	$10,000
Salvage value	$ 1,000
Total expense	$ 9,000
Life of asset	10 years
Depreciation for one year	$ 900
Depreciation for one month	$ 75

Figure 4.2. A straight-line depreciation calculation of a fixed asset.

TRANSACTIONS THAT ARE UNIQUE TO THE HEALTH CARE INDUSTRY

Contributions

Because of their not-for-profit nature and the social and charitable services they perform, hospitals receive donations of cash and other assets. The simplest form of contribution is the unrestricted donation wherein donors give cash or other assets without adding any stipulation as to how these resources are to be used. When received, this donation is recorded as revenue (the asset's fair market value is used if other than cash is received).

At times donors attach stipulations to their gifts. The hospital accepts the stipulation when it accepts this restricted donation. If the gift is restricted for activities that are within the ability of the institution, the donation is recorded as revenue upon receipt. When the donation is expended according to the donor's wishes, the expense will appear in the financial statement.

Large, restricted donations usually require separate reports that disclose how monies were used. Government grants, in particular, carry stipulations requiring federal reimbursement of any unused or improperly spent funds. Therefore, most institutions establish a restricted equity account to account for the receipt and eventual use of the funds.

Restricted donations may be made for equipment and other hospital property. These donations are also reflected as income in the period received. Their use will not result in an immediate expense because an asset has been purchased. Instead, the related expense must wait until the asset's depreciation flows through the income statement.

Donated Services

Hospitals that are operated by and use the services of members of religious orders for their daily operation may not pay these individuals a rate commensurate with the fair market value of their services. If members of a religious order are truly acting as hospital employees and receive less compensation than is paid to lay persons who perform comparable tasks, the difference between the value of the work and compensation received is labeled as donated services and listed as revenue. The full salary including the pay difference will be recorded as salary expense. This transaction will increase revenue and salary expense by the amount of the donated service and will have no impact on net income.

To be considered an employee, the service provided by the individual must be necessary to daily operation and the institution must have the right to tell the individual not only what to do, but also how and when to do it. Hospital volunteers or auxiliary workers do not satisfy the definition of hospital employee and, therefore, do not have the value of their services recorded as donated services (revenue) and salary expense.

Contractual Adjustments

Most hospitals have signed contracts with state and federal governments in which they agree to provide medical services to indigent (Medicaid) and elderly (Medicare) patients. The contracts specify that providers bill designated governmental agencies for services provided and that Medicaid and Medicare programs have agreed to pay reasonable charges for medical services. Reasonable charges are defined by each program and generally have values that are less than normal charges. (See Chapter VII for background and details.)

Hospitals charge for services based upon predetermined fee schedules. At the time of billing, the difference between billed charges and the amount that will be paid by governmental insurance providers is written off to an account called contractual adjustments. Because the difference between billed charges and reimbursable charges may not be billed to these patients, it becomes a revenue adjustment for the institution.

Bad Debts and Charity Care

Hospitals are never certain that any payment will be received. In fact, most institutions know that anywhere from four to eight percent of billed charges will not be paid by patients. Uncollectibility percentages vary greatly among health care institutions and depend upon an institution's location and the economic status of its patients.

A hospital does not know exactly which patients cannot or will not pay. Uncollectibility is generally determined after service has been provided. Most hospitals will not refuse medical service based upon a patient's inability to pay. That portion of a patient's bill that is uncollectible because of a patient's inability to pay is recorded as charity care; that portion attributable to a patient's unwillingness to pay is labeled bad debt expense. Reasons for uncollectibility are not always readily available or determinable and some overlap of charity care and bad debt expense exists. Most institutions make serious attempts to correctly identify the reason why an account is written off as uncollectible because it gives them valuable information about their economic environment and the nature of their customers. Bad debt expense is recorded as an operating expense, whereas charity care write-offs are considered a revenue adjustment.

SUMMARY

Accounting transactions occur within an institution and must be recorded, classified, summarized, and finally communicated through the financial statements. An institution develops its own timetable for recording transactions, some of which are recorded daily, weekly, or monthly.

Adjustments are needed before the financial report can be prepared because events have changed since the time the original transaction was recorded. Adjustments fall into five categories and include:

1. Recording revenue that has been earned but not yet recorded
2. Reclassifying receipts that do not represent resources that have been earned
3. Recording expenses for resources used but not paid for
4. Recording resources or inventories that have been used up
5. Recording depreciation

In addition, there are transactions that are unique to not-for-profit health care institutions. They include contributions, donated services, contractual adjustments, and charity care. All of these items affect the operations of a health care organization and must be reflected within the financial report of the entity.

QUESTIONS

1. What is the accounting cycle?
2. What determines the timing of when a transaction is recorded?
3. What are accounting adjustments? Why are adjustments needed?
4. What is depreciation? Why is an adjustment needed to record this specific item?
5. What is an unrestricted donation? How does it differ from a restricted donation? How is it reflected within the financial statements?
6. If an individual donates expertise to the institution, how should this fact be recorded? Why?

EXERCISES

Income for Hooter Hospital prior to the impact of any of the following items is reported to be $10,000. Explain how each of the following independent items will impact the balance sheet and income statement for the time period in question.

1. Salaries earned by employees but unpaid at period end totalled $500. This fact was overlooked.
2. Inventory totalling $400 was omitted from the ending physical count.
3. An annual insurance premium of $1,200 was paid at the beginning of the month and recorded as an asset. One month has expired and nothing has been recorded.
4. Patient charge slips for $200 of medical supplies were completed but omitted from the batch of charge slips that were sent to data processing.

5. Interest on $100,000 of long-term debt is due the first day of next month. Nothing has been entered to reflect one month's use of the money. Interest of 12% is charged annually.
6. A new machine costing $1,000 was expensed as a repair item. The machine has a ten-year life.
7. Employees have earned the right to $2,000 of vacation pay. This fact has not been recorded.
8. It is estimated that $1,000 of this month's patient revenue will not be collected and will have to be written off. It is unknown which accounts will be uncollectible.

V

Sample Problem

CHAPTER OBJECTIVES

1. Give a problem involving typical business transactions that occur within an accounting cycle.
2. Furnish the solution, with explanations.
3. Prepare end-of-period financial statements.

The balance sheet of Valley Hospital for the month ending January 31, 19___ appears in Figure 5.1.

Last month's balance sheet is the starting place for this month's transactions. The balance sheet shows the resources (assets) and the source of those assets. Valley has resources totalling $5,800. The creditors provided $3,500 of that total through borrowing (liabilities) and the entity has generated its own net value of $2,300 through an initial investment and earnings since its date of inception.

Instructions

The following problem has been prepared to give the reader a sense of the continuity that exists within the accounting cycle. The number of transactions and dollar amounts have been minimized so that computations will not impede understanding. Readers are asked to attempt individual transactions. The solution and its explanations are provided. It is recommended that readers identify all items involved in each transaction. Exchanges will involve the following account classifications: assets, liabilities, revenue, or expense. Revenue and expense entries should be entered directly under the equity or fund balance account, because the equity account will ultimately receive the profit or loss of the time period.

Assets		Liabilities and Fund Balance	
Cash	$ 100	Accounts Payable	$ 500
Accounts Receivable	500	Long-term Note	3,000
Inventory	400	Total Liabilities	3,500
Total Current Assets	1,000		
		Unrestricted Fund	2,300
Land	200		
Building	4,000	Total Liabilities	
Equipment	600	And Fund Balance	$5,800
	$4,800		
Total Assets	$5,800		

Figure 5.1. Valley Hospital Balance Sheet, January 31, 19__.

Current Information

The hospital prepares monthly financial statements. Below are the business transactions for the month of February, 19x0.

1. Services totalling $3,000 are provided to patients and charged to their individual patient accounts.

   Assets = Liabilities + Fund Balance

   Example: +$3,000 (Accounts Receivable) = +$3,000 (Revenue)

2. $50 of supplies are ordered and delivered, but not paid for as yet.

   Assets = Liabilities + Fund Balance

3. Patients remitted $2,500 of the amount owed on their accounts.

   Assets = Liabilities + Fund Balance

4. Equipment costing $6,000 is purchased by paying $100 and signing an agreement that calls for the remainder to be paid at the end of 6 months. A promissory note was signed for the balance owed.

   Assets = Liabilities + Fund Balance

5. Employees are paid wages totalling $1,200.

   Assets = Liabilities + Fund Balance

6. Utilities and other departmental operating expenses totalling $200 are incurred but will not be paid until next month.

   Assets = Liabilities + Fund Balance

7. Checks totalling $600 are prepared and sent to creditors.

   Assets = Liabilities + Fund Balance

8. Central Stores reports that supplies costing $300 were distributed to various departments during the month.

   Assets = Liabilities + Fund Balance

9. The hospital receives unrestricted contributions totalling $50.

   Assets = Liabilities + Fund Balance

10. Medicare pays the bill of one of its insured individuals. Medicare has sent $90 in full payment of an account that had charges totalling $100. The hospital may not bill the patient for the difference.

    Assets = Liabilities + Fund Balance

Month's-End Adjustments

11. Employees have worked 4 days since last payday, but before the end of the month. The pay for the 7-day period totals $350.

    Assets = Liabilities + Fund Balance

12. Depreciation expense for building and equipment is calculated to be $110.

    Assets = Liabilities + Fund Balance

13. Interest on the note payable is $60. Interest is owed now, but does not need to be paid until next month.

Assets = Liabilities + Fund Balance

No other adjustments were needed at month's end.

Required

Prepare the financial statements for the month of February. The financial statements include:

1. Balance Sheet
2. Income Statement
3. Statement of Changes in Fund Balance (Equity)
4. Cash Flow Statement.

(Hint: Start with the Income Statement. Then prepare the Statement of Changes in Equity, the Balance Sheet, and finally the Cash Flow Statement.)

Solution

1. Services totalling $3,000 are provided to patients and charged to their individual patient accounts.

   Explanation: The hospital has the right to future receipt of cash (asset—accounts receivable) because it provided services to patients (revenue).

Assets	= Liabilities	+	Fund Balance
+ $3,000 (Accounts Receivable) =		+	$3,000 (Revenue)

2. $50 of supplies are ordered and delivered, but have not been paid for as yet.

   Explanation: The hospital increases the asset Inventory and assumes an added liability.

Assets = Liabilities + Fund Balance
+ $50 (Supplies) = + $50 (Accounts Payable)

3. Patients paid $2,500 of the amount owed on their accounts.

Explanation: The hospital traded an asset, Accounts Receivable, and received cash.

Assets = Liabilities + Fund Balance
+ $2,500 (Cash)
- 2,500 (Accounts Receivable)
  -0- = -0- + -0-

4. Equipment costing $6,000 was purchased by paying $100 and signing an agreement that called for the balance owed to be paid at the end of 6 months. A promissory note was signed for $5,900.

Explanation: The hospital obtained the asset Equipment by giving up $100 of the asset cash and taking on an additional liability of $5,900.

Assets = Liabilities + Fund Balance
+ $6,000 (Equipment)
- 100 (Cash)
  $5,900 = + $5,900 (Note Payable)

5. Employees were paid wages totalling $1,200.

Explanation: The hospital has completely used up the services of its employees, so it is buying an expense by giving up the asset cash. Note that the employee does not receive the entire amount that has been expensed. Federal and state governments require employers to withhold from the employee's paycheck an amount for taxes that are the employee's responsibility. The amount withheld must be paid to the various governmental units and is therefore a liability to the hospital.

Assets = Liabilities + Fund Balance
- $1200 (Cash) =   - $1200 (Expense)

6. Utilities and other departmental operating expenses totalling $200 were incurred but not paid at month's end.

   Explanation: Utilities and other expenses are used up and therefore recorded as expenses. The hospital has not paid for these items, but it does have a liability to pay the various creditors.

Assets	=	Liabilities	+	Fund Balance
0	=	+ $200 (Accounts Payable)		- $200 (Expense)

7. The hospital paid $600 to its creditors.

   Explanation: The hospital is reducing its liability called Accounts Payable by reducing its Cash account.

Assets	=	Liabilities	+	Fund Balance
- $600 (Cash)	=	- $600 (Accounts Payable)		

8. Central Stores reported that supplies costing $300 were distributed to the various departments during the month.

   Explanation: The hospital uses an inventory system to identify the items used or expensed. The asset inventory should be reduced by the amount that has been used.

Assets	=	Liabilities	+	Fund Balance
- $300 (Supplies)	=			- $300 (Expense)

9. The hospital received unrestricted contributions totalling $50.

   Explanation: Cash is increased by $50. Revenue has been earned and received.

Assets	=	Liabilities	+	Fund Balance
+ $50 (Cash)	=		+	$50 (Revenue)

10. Medicare paid the bill of one of its insured individuals. They have sent $90 in full payment of an account that had charges totalling $100. The hospital may not bill the patient for the difference.

Explanation: The asset Cash is increased by $90, because the asset Accounts Receivable is decreased by $100. The difference is contractual allowance that will reduce the amount of revenue reflected on the income statement.

Assets	=	Liabilities	+	Fund Balance
+ $90 (Cash)				
- $100 (Accounts Receivable)				- $10 (Expense)
- $10	=			

The required adjusting entries are needed.

11. Employees worked 4 days since last payday but before the end of the month. The pay for the 7-day period totalled $350. Rather than calculate exactly the number of hours that were worked for those 4 days, the accountant estimates that the wages should be equal to 4/7 of the total payroll or $200. The accountant makes an adjustment to record the salary expense of the $200. Since the salary is owed and not paid, a liability for the $200 exists.

Assets	=	Liabilities	+	Fund Balance
		+ $200 (Salary Payable)		- $200 (Expense)

12. The hospital used the building and equipment during the month. Using the straight-line depreciation method, the accountant calculated the depreciation expense to be $110. Expenses are increased and the asset value is reduced through the use of the accumulated depreciation account.

Assets	=	Liabilities	+	Fund Balance
- $110 (Building and Equipment Accumulated Depreciation)				- $110 (Expense)

13. Interest on the note payable amounted to $60. Because it remains unpaid, it is a liability at month's end. The charge for interest represents an expense assessed for the use of money.

Assets	=	Liabilities	+	Fund Balance
		+ $60 (Interest Payable)		- $60 (Expense)

No other adjustments are required at month's end.

Assets		Liabilities and Fund Balance	
Cash	$ 840	Accounts Payable	$ 150
Accounts Receivable	900	Notes Payable	5,900
Supplies Inventory	150	Interest Payable	60
Total Current Assets	$1,890	Salaries Payable	200
		Total Current Liabilities	6,310
Land	$ 200	Long-term Note	$3,000
Building	4,000	Total Liabilities	$9,310
Equipment	6,600	Fund Balance	$3,270
Total Property	10,800		
Less Accumulated			
Depreciation	(110)		
	10,690		
		Total Liabilities and	
Total Assets	$12,580	Fund Balance	$12,580

Figure 5.2. Valley Hospital Balance Sheet, February 28, 19___.

Financial statements for the month ended are displayed in Figures 5.2-5.5. These statements may differ slightly from those prepared by readers. Individual account balances and classifications should be in agreement. Statement totals should also agree.

Revenue from Patient Services		$3,000
Less Medicare Contractual Adjustment		(10)
Net Patient Service Revenue		$2,990
Expenses		
Salary Expense	$1,400	
Operating	200	
Stores	300	
Depreciation	110	(2,010)
Operating Income		$ 980
Other Income/Expense		
Interest Expense	60	
Less Contribution Revenue	(50)	
Net Expense		(10)
Net Income		$ 970

Figure 5.3. Valley Hospital Income Statement for the month ending February 28, 19___.

Balance January 31, 19__	$2,300
Add income for the month	970
Balance February 28, 19__	$3,270

Figure 5.4. Valley Hospital Statement of Changes in Fund Balance, February 28, 19__.

Cash received from patients and third parties		$2,590
Cash contributions		50
Total Cash Received		$2,640
Cash paid for:		
Salaries	$1,200	
Supplies and other items	600	
		(1,800)
Cash generated by operations		840
Cash used for investments		
Purchased equipment		(6,000)
Cash received from financing		
Borrowed money to purchase equipment		5,900
Increase in cash		$ 740
Beginning cash balance		100
Cash balance February 28, 19__		$ 840

Figure 5.5. Valley Hospital Cash Flow Statement for the month ending February 28, 19__.

VI

Internal Control

CHAPTER OBJECTIVES

1. Explain the concept of internal control.
2. Explain the importance of a good system of internal control.
3. Identify characteristics of a good system of internal control.

Internal control is the system of checks and balances that exists within an institution. The purposes of a good system of internal control are:

1. To safeguard the assets of the institution
2. To ensure the generation of reliable financial information
3. To promote operational efficiency
4. To encourage adherence to management policies.[1]

A good system of internal control is essential to the financial well-being of any organization. Because its very size makes it impossible for the chief executive officer to supervise or perform all of the many tasks that are necessary to keep an institution operating, delegation must take place. It becomes necessary for managers at every level to delegate tasks while retaining responsibility for their completion. Internal control is the name given to the system that incorporates check points and specific review procedures into ongoing activities. The primary purposes of internal control are to safeguard the assets and to generate reliable financial records.

There are specific control features that an organization can build into its operating structure to strengthen internal control. They include, but are not limited to, the following:

1. Definition of lines of authority
2. Definition and documentation of employee duties
3. Separation of strategic duties
4. Use of formal, written documentation
5. Use of written authorization and approval mechanisms at important intervals or processes
6. Use of machines to document transactions
7. Restriction of access to easily appropriated assets
8. Rotation of employee duties within a department
9. Use of external auditors
10. Creation of an internal auditing department

These features are explained in further detail throughout the remainder of this chapter.

Definition of the Lines of Authority

A hospital should have an organizational chart that is formally prepared and distributed to all departments. This organizational chart should clarify existing lines of authority that connect the chief executive officer to the departments. In this way, employees know to whom and for whom they are responsible. Besides defining lines of authority and responsibility, an organizational chart also identifies the formal communication network that links all facets of an organization to its chief executive officer.

Definition and Documentation of Employee Duties

In addition to the organizational chart, every employee position or job category should be documented. A job description should outline assigned tasks that an employee is expected to perform during his or her workday. It should also identify the position to which the employee reports. Its existence and use will prevent errors of commission and/or omission.

Separation of Duties

As an institution grows in size, more personnel are added to its work force. As numbers of employees increase, a division of duties can be incorporated into daily work routines. One safety feature of a good system of internal control is a separation of crucial financial functions, such as receiving cash and making payments, ordering, receiving, and/or using goods. By separating critical functions into different tasks performed by different individuals or sometimes by different departments, each individual or department is able to review the work performed by others. Each review procedure reduces the risk of an error occurring and remaining undetected. It also guards against assets being misdirected, misappropriated, or wasted.

Use of Formal, Written Documentation

Written records should be prepared and maintained as records of business transactions. Whenever possible, preprinted forms should be used to identify information needed and to facilitate the recording process. Written documentation furnishes interested parties with an opportunity to review all supporting details of transactions. It also furnishes proof that a business transaction has occurred, while allowing others a chance to reconstruct what happened, identify all parties involved in the transaction, and ascertain that it was properly authorized and recorded.

Important documents such as checks, purchase orders, and invoices should be preprinted and prenumbered. Periodically, prenumbered documents should be checked and all numbers accounted for.

Use of Written Authorization and Approval

A good system of internal control should specify those functions that are within the jurisdiction of each individual (as documented in the job description). As individuals perform their assigned tasks, they should record that fact by noting or initialing what work has been finished. Thus, a decision or an event is assured of being recorded. Supervisors should regularly review sign-off procedures to ensure adherence to established policies.

As transactions increase in importance, more approvals and authorizations should be required for each transaction. For example, it may take only one person to approve a purchase order that amounts to less then $5,000; while two or more individuals may be required to authorize a purchase of more than that amount. Approvals and authorizations should be permanently recorded. They are then available and subject to review by the other managers and auditors.

Use of Machines to Document Transactions

Many organizations use machines to record data, especially when there are many quantitative transactions. For example, many use time clocks to record employee arrivals and departures. Employees punch in because they know that in order to receive payment for time worked, their hours must be visibly recorded on time cards. Supervisors review and initial time cards to ensure that the system records only those hours worked. This procedure takes time but it increases control because supervisors may catch employee omissions or improper recordings. Exceptions, such as sick time, vacation, or overtime, can be approved and verified immediately.

Cash registers are another example of machines that are used to record business transactions. Employees who receive cash must record those receipts in a cash register so that a machine-generated receipt can be produced. Individuals tendering money expect to receive this receipt. At the same time that a receipt is prepared, that transaction is recorded on a duplicate paper tape inside the machine. Once recorded, the information is trapped inside the machine and cannot be changed. At the end of the day, the cash register prints out totals of that day's transactions.

Restriction of Access to Easily Appropriated Assets

As a continuation of the previous example, money in a cash drawer must agree with its machine printout. To ensure that this machine strengthens internal control, an institution must provide that only one person is assigned to a machine between those times when totals are printed out, and that the keys that open the cash registers are held by supervisors who do not operate them.

Rotation of Employee Duties

Employees should replace each other during vacation and other absences. Replacement employees can then review current operating procedures. Errors and/or discrepancies can be detected. Rotation of employee duties will also provide new employees with a fresh perspective and an opportunity to review the operation. Suggestions for different time- and/or cost-saving procedures may result. If an absent employee had been performing a task incorrectly, the replacement should discover this fact. In conjunction with this feature, employees, especially those who handle cash, should be required to take their annual vacations.

Use of External Auditors

Many organizations engage independent certified public accountants to audit financial records and to give an opinion as to the fairness of the financial statements.

External auditors review and test internal control. They also perform tests and auditing procedures that are designed to reaffirm financial data and to detect material errors and discrepancies if they exist within the financial data. Auditors may correspond directly with patients to confirm their individual account balances. Auditors may also observe hospital employees taking physical inventory of central stores and pharmacy. There are many other auditing tests that external auditors perform to satisfy themselves that financial information is properly recorded and fairly presented.

External auditors are independent of the entity itself. It is because of this independence that an auditor's opinion is highly valued.

Creation of an Internal Auditing Department

An organization may be large enough to justify an internal audit department. Internal auditing's purpose is to continuously review internal control and operations. Internal auditors review and test operating efficiency and departmental adherence to management policies. They perform tests to ensure that assets are safeguarded and that reliable financial records are generated. The role of internal auditor is more inclusive and pervasive than that of external auditor. Internal auditors are employees of the organization, but are independent of the departments they audit. Theirs is a continuous review operation, whereas external auditors test and review year-end financial statements and overall operations.

Drawbacks to Any System of Internal Control

Any system of internal control has its own inherent limitations. Even the best system will not always function properly. Generally, system malfunctions are caused by human error, either intentional or unintentional. Errors may result from poor training, carelessness, fatigue, errors in judgment, or intentional fraudulent acts. A good system of internal control should identify and correct human errors and detect fraudulent activity before they are permanently recorded.

There may be occasions when part of the system breaks down. Any discrepancy that is found should be investigated immediately. Discrepancies may be intentional. Consequently, system irregularities should be investigated immediately. The nature and extent of errors must be determined so that steps can be taken to correct the situation.

Apparently isolated situations should be documented and corrected. Similar past transactions should be reviewed to ascertain that this is an isolated instance. If a recurring error is found, prior transactions need verification to correct its effects. Reasons for errors must be determined to identify contributing factors that led to and could continue to cause further breakdowns.

SUMMARY

The system of internal control that is incorporated into operations is designed to protect entity assets, to ensure that reliable financial information is recorded and transmitted, and to promote operational efficiency and internal adherence to management policies. There are many control features that can be incorporated into daily procedures to accomplish these goals.

REFERENCES ─────────────────────────────

1. American Institute of Certified Public Accountants, *AICPA Professional Standards,* Vol. 1. Auditing Section AU Sec. 320.10. New York, 1988.

QUESTIONS ─────────────────────────────

1. What is internal control?
2. What is the purpose of a good system of internal control?
3. Why is a good system of internal control necessary to the financial well-being of an entity?
4. What are some of the methods that an entity can use to improve its system of internal control?
5. Should an entity incorporate all of the features of a good system of internal control into its operating procedures? What considerations should be addressed before implementing changes to any system?
6. What is meant by cost benefit analysis? Why is it important to use this analysis when drafting procedures that are designed to strengthen internal control?
7. What are inherent drawbacks to any system of internal control? What can be done to overcome them? Can they ever be completely eliminated?
8. If an error or weakness in internal control is identified, what should be done?

EXERCISES ─────────────────────────────

For each of the following situations, identify the internal control features that the business has incorporated into its operations.

1. Purchases that are returned to a retail store must have a return slip prepared before money can be refunded. The return slip must be approved by the department supervisor before money can be given.
2. When purchasing gasoline from the local self-serve station, the individual uses a pump that measures the amount and retail value of gasoline purchased.

3. Supply requisitions must be filled out and approved by a designated department before an order will be placed.
4. Employees receive their wages in the form of a payroll check. The payroll check is prenumbered.
5. Each employee in the department has specific assigned responsibilities.
6. Narcotics and other medical supplies are kept in a locked or restricted area. It may be necessary to sign for any items that are taken from this area.
7. Charge slips for ordered laboratory procedures are sent to the laboratory to initiate the procedure. The charge slips are then sent to data processing for billing.
8. Patients and their insurance carriers are mailed detailed statements of tests and services that were provided to the patient.
9. A separate listing of tests, their results, and physician's and nurse's progress reports are sent to and filed with medical records.
10. An employee terminating service with an institution will have an exit routine in which keys are returned, reasons for leaving are ascertained, and the employee's final payroll check is picked up.

CASE

You are responsible for patients on a medical unit. One patient has been on the unit for three days. You know that the patient is uninsured and does not have the money to pay his bill. A student nurse has come to you and suggested that medical supplies be given to this patient without processing any charge slips. The student feels that it is a waste of time, both yours and data processing's, to process charges that cannot be collected. How should you answer the student nurse? Discuss what should be done. Explain your answer.

VII

The Economic and Legal Environment of the Health Care Industry

CHAPTER OBJECTIVES

1. Trace the economic changes in the environment of the health care industry.
2. Identify the financial impact of specific health care legislation.
   - A. Title XVIII and Title XIX
   - B. Minimum Wage Laws
   - C. Economic Stabilization Act of 1970
   - D. PL 92-603
   - E. PL 93-541, Health Planning and Resource Development Act of 1974
   - F. PL 97-248 Tax Equity and Fiscal Responsibility Act of 1982 (TEFRA)
3. Identify other economic factors that have had an impact upon the health care delivery system.

If it were possible to return to 1965 and compare hospitals of that period to those of today, readers would be impressed by the much simpler internal structures of yesterday's institutions. Accounting departments would have been insignificant units, whose primary purpose was preparing financial statements. That task would have been performed by bookkeepers and the various internal functions of general accounting, accounts payable, and payroll would have been consolidated under one department head. These departments could have been staffed with less than 10 employees.

Even then, patients' accounts was a separate department, whose primary responsibility was accumulating patient charges, preparing third-party bills, and collecting patient account balances. It was before the advent of computers, and bookkeepers manually recorded transactions using simple bookkeeping machines.

The majority of hospitals were and still are organized as not-for-profit corporations, founded by communities, religious orders, or governmental bodies. Figure 7.1 shows the number of hospitals in operation in 1960, 1970, and 1980, by ownership. Inpatient service generated 90% of revenue, and patients and insurance carriers paid full charges. Hospitals generated sufficient revenue to cover their relatively low operating expenses, and private contributions covered any operating deficits that occurred.

Since those good old days, many things have drastically changed the health care environment. Titles XVIII and XIX Amendments to the Social Security Act were passed in 1965 and reimbursement under this legislation was fully implemented by 1968. Even before reimbursement rules were defined, the federal government circulated contracts to any interested party. Most hospitals signed these contracts agreeing to provide services to program patients and to bill the government agencies for services rendered.

Title XVIII offers medical insurance to the nation's elderly, giving them access to the nation's health care delivery system. Any individual who is eligible for retirement benefits under Social Security is also entitled to health care coverage under Title XVIII (Medicare). This insurance umbrella is funded by the FICA (Social Security) taxes that are levied on and deducted from employee wages and matched by employer contributions. Title XIX (Medicaid) is an insurance policy for the indigent. It is administered by individual state governments, and funded with both state and federal money.

Initial legislation provided insurance coverage, but did not specify how reimbursement would be effected other than saying that health care providers would be paid "reasonable charges" for services provided. All general reimbursement guidelines are developed under the auspices of the Department of Health and Human Services (formerly the Department of Health, Education and Welfare) which established the Health Care Financing Administration (HCFA) to develop specific forms and procedures (Health Insurance Manual 15—HIM 15).

"Reasonable charges" were initially interpreted to mean actual incurred costs plus a minimal 2% profit added. Medicare and Medicaid

	1960	**1970**	**1980**
Not-for-profit	3,291	3,386	3,350
Owner invested (for-profit)	856	769	727
Federal	435	408	361
State/local government	1,260	1,704	1,846
All hospitals	6,876	7,123	6,988

Figure 7.1. Ownership of hospitals, 1960, 1970, 1980.

began reimbursing providers under this cost-plus arrangement. HCFA identified those costs that are allowable under the program. Bad debts and charity care were the first expenses to be disallowed. From its inception, Medicare included patient-pay provisions for deductibles and coinsurance. These amounts are billed directly to patients. Medicare reimburses bad debts only to the extent that program patients fail to pay their deductibles and coinsurance. In later years, malpractice insurance premiums and self-insurance programs were largely excluded from reimbursement.

Determining costs associated with providing patient services is difficult. HIM 15 outlines a cost report that accumulates costs and allocates service department costs to revenue producing units. Program patient bills were reimbursed retrospectively using a ratio of charges to charges applied to costs. Most states have also adopted this cost report format for Medicaid reimbursement.

Example

If the nonrevenue-producing department to be allocated is laundry, its allocation basis would be pounds of clean laundry distributed. For simplicity, assume that there are only two other hospital departments. Direct departmental costs have already been totalled. Activity data (pounds of clean laundry distributed) has been gathered for all other departments. Figure 7.2 depicts the cost allocation calculations to arrive at the total cost associated with Surgery and Laboratory. Figure 7.3 further applies the principles of RCCAC (rate of covered charges to accumulated costs) to total costs to arrive at Medicare reimbursement. The initial years of reimbursement included a 2% profit element.

	Cost Centers			Total
	Laundry	**Surgery**	**Lab**	
Pounds of linen used		9,000	1,000	10,000
Departmental costs	$6,000	$40,000	$20,000	$66,000
Cost/pound of linen* ($0.60)				
Allocated laundry costs	($6,000)			
to Surgery**		$ 5,400		
to Laboratory***			$ 600	
Total department costs	–0–	$45,400	$20,600	$66,000

*$6,000 divided by 10,000 lbs.
** 9,000 lbs. at $.60
***(1,000 lbs. at $.60)

Figure 7.2.   Cost allocation under RCCAC.

	Surgery	Laboratory
Medicare Revenue	$20,000	$25,000
Total Departmental Revenue	$80,000	$50,000
Medicare Utilization Rate	25%	50%
Reimbursable costs		
Department costs*	$45,400	$20,600
Medicare's Share**	$11,350	$10,300
Initial Profit Allocation (2%)	$ 227	$ 206
Total Reimbursement	$11,577	$10,506

*From Figure 7.2
**Departmental costs multiplied by Medicare utilization rate.

Figure 7.3.   Application of RCCAC principles to total costs to derive Medicare reimbursement.

Cost Center or Department	Base
Depreciation — Building and Equipment	Square Footage
Employee Benefits	Gross Salaries
General and Administrative Expenses	Accumulated Costs
Maintenance and Repairs	Square Footage
Operation of the Plant	Square Footage
Laundry	Pounds of Clean Linen used
Housekeeping	Hours of service
Dietary	Meals served
Cafeteria	Meals served to employees
Maintenance of personnel	Number of employees housed
Nursing Administration	Hours of service, nurses
Central Service	Costed Requisitions
Pharmacy	Costed Requisitions
Medical Records and Library	Time Spent
Nursing School	Assigned time of nurses
Interns and Residents	Assigned time

Figure 7.4. Allocation bases for nonrevenue-producing departments.

Similar allocations would be performed on other nonrevenue-producing departments until all costs are borne by the revenue producers. Figure 7.4 provides a listing of the nonrevenue-producing departments and their RCCAC allocation base. Using RCCAC, the Medicare utilization is calculated by department and applied to total accumulated costs.

There is a great deal of record keeping involved in preparing cost reports. Statistics must be accurately maintained to support cost allocations. Each program also requires maintenance of patient logs detailing patient name, admission number, total inpatient days, and billed charges for each revenue-producing department. Separate patient logs and charges are also maintained for program outpatients.

All reports and records are subject to external audit. HCFA selects intermediaries, generally local Blue Cross Hospital Insurance plans, to oversee daily billing and reimbursement procedures and to act on their behalf. Reimbursement is handled in a manner similar to individual income tax withholdings. Using patient bills as the basis for initial reimbursement, intermediaries pay fees based upon their schedule (prior to 1987, a percentage of billed charges; after 1987, based on DRG (diagnostic related group) fees). Before 1987, final inpatient and outpatient reimbursement settlements were made at year end as a result of the cost report. Any difference between reimbursable program costs and interim payments resulted in a final settlement balance to be paid or received by providers.

Nursing Differential

As Medicare costs escalated, legislation was passed to cut provider reimbursement. In 1970, the 2% profit element was replaced with an 8 1/2% nursing differential charge that increased the reimbursement of nursing costs only. The cost reimbursement of other ancillary departments remained unchanged. For example, if the hospital's average cost per patient day is $100, Medicare's charge per patient day was $108.50.

Public Law 92-603

In 1972, Congress passed PL 92-603 which stated that Medicare and Medicaid would pay the lesser of costs or billed charges. Congress believed that since hospitals were generally not-for-profit institutions, they should not receive a profit for providing services to elderly and indigent patients. Congress stated that hospitals should be given only the cost of providing the service. In cases where costs were greater than billed charges, reimbursement was limited to billed charges.

PL 92-603 further established cost limitations under Section 223. This section established hospital group classifications based upon geographic region and institution size. Reimbursement was limited to a specified percentage applied to the average cost of an individual hospital's group. Providers competed with each other and high-cost providers were unable to recoup all of their costs for providing services. Their choices were to cease providing services to program patients, suffer losses, or reduce costs.

Medicare Intermediaries

Because the Department of Health and Human Services and the Health Care Financing Administration did not want to be involved with the intricacies of reimbursement, they selected third-party intermediaries for each state to act on their behalf. In the beginning, the role of intermediaries was undefined, leaving some to act as hospital advocates and others as hospital adversaries. Each intermediary ruling affected provider reimbursement and rulings were based upon each intermediary's interpretation of HIM-15. Intermediary rulings lacked consistency from state to state, or, within a state, from year to year. Interpretations of one period were not binding on other periods.

The Provider Reimbursement Review Board (PRRB) was established to alleviate some of these inconsistencies and seemingly arbitrary intermediary decisions. Its function was to settle reimbursement disputes that arose between providers and their intermediaries. The PRRB soon became inundated with provider disputes and was required to establish a minimum cost limit of $10,000.

Financial Implications of Medicare and Medicaid Legislation

Because of the added data-gathering, cost-finding, and reimbursement requirements of Titles XVIII and XIX, hospitals were forced to replace bookkeepers with financial managers. A staff of accountants was hired to realign fee structures. In many cases, they also had to establish mechanisms to identify and accumulate departmental costs, revenues, and activity statistics. Financial managers had to struggle to understand HIM-15 instructions. Once understood, several interim cost reports had to be prepared to ensure that departmental costs were in line with departmental charges. New fees had to be calculated and established for those departments that charged less than the costs of providing the service. Financial managers had to anticipate the financial effects that new services and program amendments would have on cost allocations and program reimbursement.

The number of patient account billing clerks in the patient accounts department increased due to the patient logs that had to be maintained. Also, Medicare or Medicaid processed only their own long, complex billing forms. The billing problem has been rectified somewhat because HCFA implemented a national, uniform billing (HCFA-1450), but not until 1984.

Minimum Wage Law

Until 1967, hospital employees were exempted from coverage by the Minimum Wage Law because their employees did not engage in inter-

	Before	After
Pay Classification	1967	1967
Attendant	$1.25	$1.60
Staff Nurse	$3.00	$3.80
Technician	$2.00	$2.50

Figure 7.5. The ripple effect on wages.

state commerce. In 1967, a special amendment to the Minimum Wage Law expressly included hospital employees under this legislation, raising the lowest hourly wage base to $1.60 an hour. Since an increase in the hourly rate of the lowest pay class alone would destroy the equity of an institution's wage scale structure, most hospitals were forced to raise the hourly rates of all of the various employee pay classifications. This created a ripple effect (see Figure 7.5).

As a result of inclusion under the Minimum Wage Law, salaries increased by as much as 25% to 30%; this in an industry that was and continues to be highly labor-intensive (approximating 70% of total hospital costs).

Economic Stabilization Act

During the 1970s, the effects of prolonged inflation were being felt by all aspects of the economy. In an attempt to curb inflation, President Nixon signed the Economic Stabilization Act. Its effect was to freeze all wages and prices. After approximately eight months, President Nixon lifted wage and price restrictions from all industries except health care. Under continued legislation, health care was permitted an overall increase of 6% in patient revenues. The 6% increase was computed on base period fees that existed just prior to the "freeze."

Health care was singled out for continued restrictions because the rate of increase in health care costs was almost three times that of the Gross National Product. Health care was viewed as playing a major role in spiraling inflation.

Since approximately 70% of a hospital's costs were for labor, a wage increase of 4.2% of base period wages was allowed. The remaining 30% of costs were spent for nonwage expenses. These expenses were allowed to increase 1.8% over base costs.

All other manufacturers of goods and services were allowed to increase their prices by any rate that they desired. Wages of employees in non-health care industries were increased without restriction. The 6% price restriction was maintained on health care alone.

Even though hospitals purchased supplies from outsiders who increased their prices more than 1.8%, hospitals could only pass on a 1.8% fee increase to its patients. The result was that most hospitals suffered operating losses during this period. Several were even forced into bankruptcy.

Within a year, wage and price restrictions were lifted from hospitals. One expert projected that "if the price controls had been kept on hospitals for another two or three years, hundreds, maybe thousands, of hospitals would have gone bankrupt."[1]

The Economy

The technological boom also contributed to the rising cost of health care. In part a by-product of the space program, this boom brought new and more sophisticated equipment, as well as new medical and surgical techniques, to the public. Accident victims and cancer and heart patients benefitted from this research. The cost of new equipment and the wages of the skilled technicians who were needed to operate the equipment were high, but every hospital sought to purchase the latest "state of the art" machines, primarily because staff physicians and the general public required it. In many instances, newly acquired equipment was made obsolete shortly after it was delivered. The constant push to improve technology kept hospitals buying and leasing newer and better equipment, causing dramatic increases in health care costs. Add to this the impact that insuring the elderly and the indigent had on increased hospital utilization, and it is no wonder that health care costs were a constant focus of attention. Figure 7.6 provides a listing of dollars spent on health care and relates these to total gross national product for the years listed. Titles XVIII and XIX budgets were grossly underestimated. This was due in part to uncertainty regarding patient utilization, and in part to program patients' prolonged life due to continued use of the health care system. "Older people are subject to more disability, see physicians 50% more often and have twice as many hospital stays that last almost twice as long as is true of younger persons. The aged represent 10% of the population and 29% of the health care expenditures."[2]

Congress responded to Medicare and Medicaid programs' increased costs by first increasing employee FICA taxes. FICA taxes can be increased in one of three ways: by increasing 1) the tax rate, 2) its

Year	Billions of Dollars	As % of GNP	Public Payment as % of Total
1950	12.7	4.4	22. 0
1955	17.7	4.4	22. 6
1960	26.9	5.3	20. 8
1965	41.7	6.0	21. 0
1970	74.7	7.5	33. 4
1975	132.7	8.6	38. 5
1980	247.2	9.4	39. 2

Figure 7.6. National health care expenditures, as a percentage of gross national product.

taxable base, or 3) both. Figure 7.7 recaps the rapid changes in the annual FICA tax structure.

Medical Deductibles and Coinsurance

Congress attempted to reduce its portion of Medicare health care costs by shifting some of the payment burden to the patient. A deductible of $52 per event (an event is considered to be one inpatient stay per 60-day period) was included in the initial Medicare insurance coverage. In 1987, that deductible was increased to $520 per event.

Congress also increased coinsurance rates from $13 a day for patient stays in excess of 60 days in one year to $130 a day. Even with these increased patient pay elements, Medicare continued to operate at a deficit.

Congress cut reimbursable costs by first decreasing the nursing differential payment from 8 1/2% to 5%. In an attempt to curtail duplicity of service, Congress signed PL 93-541, Health Planning and Resource Development Act of 1974, which established Health Systems Agencies. This act established area planning councils who review petitions for changes in bed complements (either increases or decreases) and new equipment purchases costing more than $150,000 (later increased to $600,000 as the result of the Omnibus Budget Reconciliation Act of 1981). Each hospital requesting a change in number of beds or acquisition of equipment with a price greater than the threshold is required to file a certificate of need (CON). The area planning council reviews this and decides whether requested changes are necessary. If a

Year	Tax Rate	Taxable Base	Employee Tax Paid
1965	3.625%	$ 4,800	$ 174
1970	4.4	7,800	374
1975	5.2	14,100	733
1980	6.13	25,900	1,588
1985	7.05	39,600	2,792
1990	7.85	50,300	3,948

Figure 7.7. FICA tax rate increases over time.*

petition is granted, a provider may make the necessary expenditures, passing interest and depreciation costs on to Medicare and Medicaid. If a petition is denied, the hospital is supposed to abide by the decision of the council and refrain from purchasing these items. The system is entirely voluntary. If a hospital ignores a negative council decision and purchases equipment or changes bed complement, related interest and depreciation costs become disallowed costs.

Area planning councils have not been able to restrict capital expenditures. In many instances they have become political instruments and are often bogged down with bureaucratic procedures. Often it is only a matter of time before the CON is granted. As a result of its inefficiency, several states have stopped funding these councils.*

Tax Equity and Fiscal Responsibility Act of 1982

In 1982, Congress passed the Tax Equity and Fiscal Responsibility Act of 1982—Public Law 97-248 (TEFRA). TEFRA established target charge rates based upon the inpatient case mix that the hospital served during the year. The International Classification of Diseases—9th Revision—Clinical Modification (ICD-9-CM) was adopted as the basis of coding inpatient cases. This coding scheme permits classification of patient diseases, first into 23 categories by body organ and then into

* From *Prentice Hall Tax Guide*. Prentice Hall Publishers, New York, 1990. Par. 34,874.

467 diagnostic related groups (DRGs), based upon medical and surgical procedures performed.

DRG cost analysis was first utilized by TEFRA to establish retrospective cost limits. These cost screens were then applied to provider cost reports to establish maximum reimbursement levels.

Social Security Amendments

The Social Security Amendments of 1983 (Public Law 98-21) established a prospective reimbursement schedule based upon DRGs. The goal of the DRG system is to establish a fee schedule using national average case costs to be phased in over a 4+ year period. In the first year, the per case reimbursement comprised 75% actual hospital costs and 25% national average cost. In the second year, it changed to 50% hospital costs, 50% national average costs. For the third year, the target split is 25% individual hospital costs and 75% national average costs. By the end of the fourth year, reimbursement is expected to be 100% national average costs.

Under prospective payment systems using DRGs, reimbursement rates are established by diagnosis at the beginning of each year. The diagnosis at admission is modified by four additional diagnoses (if needed) and three procedures, with adjustments made for patient age, sex, and discharge status. Not all costs are included in the DRG base. Capital related costs (fixed asset depreciation and interest), certain professional education program costs, graduate medical education costs, and compensation of hospital-based physicians continue to be reimbursed retrospectively using cost report information. National DRGs are also adjusted for differences in local wage components, thus making them somewhat area-specific.

The following providers are excluded from the prospective payment system:

1. Psychiatric hospitals
2. Rehabilitation hospitals
3. Children's hospitals
4. Qualifying cancer hospitals
5. Hospitals with an average patient stay of greater than 25 days

All of these institutions remain subject to TEFRA limitations. Outpatient services are also reimbursed under the retrospective cost reporting system.

The prospective payment system provides reduced cost reimbursement for individual patients who fall outside the normal statistics. Referred to as "outliers," these cases receive additional but not full payment for services rendered.

Other Economic Changes

Malpractice insurance has greatly added to health care cost over the past two decades. Because annual insurance premiums have increased by as much as 500% during that period, many institutions cannot afford to fully insure themselves and have accepted deductibles of $1 million or more.

During the last two decades, the health care industry has seen a definite departure from admitting and treating patients in-house. Utilization of outpatient services has increased dramatically in response to utilization review and the ever-increasing costs of inpatient services. The volume of outpatient service has also increased in response to the highly competitive marketplace. Individual hospitals must offer services that are available at other hospitals or local ambulatory care facilities. Patients demand more services and convenient times and locations.

More emphasis is being placed on preventive medicine by emphasizing good nutrition, exercise, and regular checkups. Hospitals are entering the patient education arena, offering seminars on topics such as weight loss and breaking the smoking habit. Hospitals continue to expand their market perspective. This is evidenced by the emergence of hospital-sponsored home health agencies, nursing homes, and health maintenance organizations. Still other institutions are building satellite ambulatory care centers in outlying neighborhoods.

Hospitals must compete with other industries for employees and supplies. Employee salaries have increased to remain competitive and ensure that sufficient, qualified employees are available to satisfy present and future needs. Inflation and the need for specialized services have kept salaries a major cost of doing business.

SUMMARY

Legislation has continued to reduce hospital reimbursement for Medicare and Medicaid program patients, at the same time that inflation and technological boom are forcing health care costs upward. Health care costs continue to increase at a faster rate than does the Gross National Product. This rate of increase has pushed the health care industry into the spotlight and subjected it to constant political, media, and public scrutiny.

Hospitals must employ shrewd financial managers to survive. Efficient business practices must be formulated and communicated to all levels of management bringing cost containment to all employees.

REFERENCES

[1]Donald F. Beck, *Basic Hospital Financial Management,* Aspen Systems Corporation, Rockville, Maryland. 1980. p . 2.
[2]Ibid., p.2.

QUESTIONS

1. Discuss the impact that Title XVIII and Title XIX have had on reimbursement.
2. What are the indirect costs associated with Medicare and Medicaid?
3. What is the logic that supports a reimbursement system that is other than billed charges?
4. What role do deductibles and coinsurance play in reimbursement?
5. Why was the Economic Stabilization Act especially unfair to the health care industry?
6. What is the impact of the trends in legislation as they affect the health care industry? Do you agree with them? Discuss what alternatives may be available to the industry.
7. What impact did TEFRA have upon the health care industry?
8. What is the difference between retrospective and prospective reimbursement? Would hospital management policies differ depending upon which form of reimbursement was in place?

SECTION *II*

Operation and Management

VIII

The Nature of Costs

Hospital departments incur costs as part of daily operations. These costs vary over time as departmental operating levels change from month to month, reflecting different patient and physician demands for services. There are basic cost behavior patterns that may exist between activity levels and accumulated costs. Managers with knowledge of specific departmental cost behavior patterns have the insight needed to predict, monitor, and control costs.

As departmental activity increases, some, but not necessarily all, department costs increase. To understand a department more fully, managers must identify the cost/activity relationships that exist within each department.

Two basic cost/activity relationships exist and are referred to as fixed and variable. The fixed cost/activity relationship exists when an item's total cost does not vary as activity levels change. Variable cost describes an item whose cost increases proportionately as the level of

Month	Head Nurse Salary A	Patient Days B	Cost/Patient Day A /B
May	$2,000	450	$4.55
June	$2,000	420	$4.76
July	$2,000	540	$3.70

Figure 8.1. Fixed cost per activity unit.

activity increases, or decreases proportionately as the activity level decreases. Each cost behavior pattern is explained more fully in this text.

Fixed Costs

Fixed costs are period costs (costs that are associated with a period of time rather than an activity) whose total amount remains unchanged even though activity levels change from one time period to the next. The salary of a nursing supervisor is an example of a fixed cost. A nursing supervisor's salary remains unchanged regardless of the unit's level of occupancy. There can be 15, 18, 20, or more patients in residence on a nursing unit and the head nurse draws the same pay.

While total cost remains constant, the cost per activity unit fluctuates with its changes. When work or activity increases, the cost per work unit decreases. Conversely, when activity decreases, the cost per work unit increases. For example, a 20-bed nursing unit with one head nurse whose salary is $2,000 per month might use patient days as its activity unit. If patient days for May, June, and July are 450, 420, and 540, respectively, the head nurse cost per patient day is $4.55, $4.76, and $3.70, respectively (see Figure 8.1 for details).

The greater the level of activity (total patient days), the lower the fixed cost associated with each patient day. Therefore, as activity increases, total fixed costs remain constant, but the fixed cost per unit decreases. Conversely, as departmental activity decreases, total fixed costs remain unchanged, causing an increase in per unit cost. See Figure 8.2 for a graph depicting fixed costs.

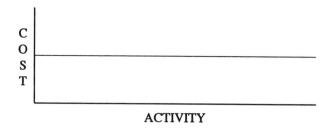

ACTIVITY

Figure 8.2. Fixed costs.

Variable Costs

A variable cost is one that varies directly with the level of activity because the cost per unit of activity remains constant. Therefore, as activity levels increase, total variable cost increases, and when activity levels decrease, total variable cost decreases. The cost increase or decrease changes in direct proportion to the change in the activity level. If supply expense is variable, the detail information for total costs should approximate the cost behavior pattern exhibited in Figure 8.3.

In reality, cost/activity relationships are not exact, but approximate a variable or a fixed cost pattern. Very few cost categories maintain a constant variable cost per unit. Reasons for minor differences include item price changes, inflation, technological improvements, quantity discounts, uneven usage, and waste. A graph of the variable cost behavior pattern can be seen in Figure 8.4.

Month	Supply Cost A	Patient Days B	Cost/Patient Day A / B
May	$900	450	$2
June	$840	420	$2
July	$1,080	540	$2

Figure 8.3. Cost behavior for variable cost.

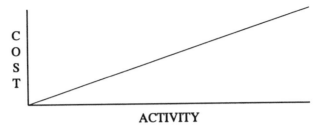

Figure 8.4. Variable cost behavior pattern.

Mixed Costs

Fixed and variable cost patterns are the most basic cost/activity relationships that exist. Specific costs or charges are accumulated in expense accounts and then summarized in monthly financial statements. An organization adopts a classification methodology that labels expenses under titles such as salaries, supplies, and other. A specific cost category such as salaries expense may have fixed and variable cost components included in the one account. If it does, the expense is referred to as a mixed cost.

Utilities expense is an example of a mixed cost because there will be some heat, light, and power used by nursing units even if there are no patients being treated there. The cost associated with the minimum required power usage is the fixed cost component. As the level of activity increases and more inpatient and outpatient services are provided, power usage increases, adding to the utility bill. That portion of the bill associated with activity changes is its variable cost component. A manager needs to separate a mixed cost into its fixed and variable components to understand and control a department's operating costs. There are several methods that can be used to isolate fixed and variable costs, some more sophisticated and complex than others.

Graphing Mixed Costs

Plotting various costs associated with various monthly activity levels may help a manager identify cost behavior patterns. After monthly cost/activity points have been plotted, a manager should try to fit a straight line through the center of these points. The point where the line intersects the "x" or vertical axis marks the fixed cost component of the mixed cost. The variable cost component can be isolated by noting the slope of the line which identifies amount of change that

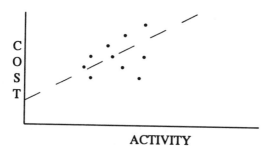

Figure 8.5. Scatter diagram used to isolate fixed and variable cost components.

occurs in the total cost due to increased units of activity. Figure 8.5 illustrates the graphing method used to isolate fixed and variable cost components. The graph shows a fixed cost component approximating $1,500 and a variable cost component that is close to $1.00 per unit.

Scatter diagrams are simple to prepare and understand, and they do display whether a relationship exists. The cluster of points also displays the degree of change within the relationship. However, scatter diagrams often lack exactness because they rely on their makers' ability to draw a straight line through a series of plotted points, and then interpret the results. To do this properly, a relationship must exist, and the diagram must be drawn to scale, a feat that cannot always be accomplished. Finally, not all mixed cost behaviors can be plotted by using a straight line. There are some cost behaviors that are curvilinear. This is because the variable cost per unit decreases as the level of activity increases due to increased user efficiency or volume purchase discounts.

Despite its disadvantages, graphing's simplicity and ability to display the degree to which cost/activity relationships exist for a given department make it a viable management tool. The extent to which it can be used to identify fixed and variable cost components of a mixed cost depends upon the specific relationship and an individual's ability to capture that information pictorially.

High/Low Method — Mixed Costs

The high/low method can be used to separate the fixed and variable cost components of a mixed cost. It calculates these components using the cost and activity information associated with the highest and lowest activity periods.

Month	Cost	Activity
January	$10,500	200
February	$13,200	260
March	$ 9,800	180
April	$11,566	209
May	$13,000	243

Figure 8.6. Activity and cost by month.

An example of the high/low method appears in Figure 8.6. The first step in the process is to identify the highest (February, $13,200/260) and lowest cost/activity month (March, $9,800/180). All other data and months are ignored. The next step is to subtract data (cost and activity) related to the low period from that of the high period, as in Figure 8.7 ($13,200 – $9,800 = $3,400; 260 – 180 = 80).

The difference in cost should be due entirely to its variable cost component because, by definition, fixed costs will not change with activity changes. Since $3,400 represents the cost associated with performing the additional 80 units of work, the variable cost per unit of work is $42.50 ($3,400 divided by 80). By substituting the variable cost per unit into a formula for February's total cost, the fixed component can be isolated (see Figure 8.8).

Month	Cost	Activity
February	$13,200	260
March	– 9,800	– 180
Difference	$ 3,400	80
Variable cost per unit = $3,400 ÷ 80 or $42.50		

Figure 8.7. Solving for the variable cost per unit.

Y		a	+	bX	
Total Cost	=	Fixed Cost	+	Variable Cost	
$13,200	=	Fixed Cost	+	260 units @ $42.50/unit	
$13,200	=	Fixed Cost	+	$11,050	
$ 2,150	=	Fixed Cost			

Figure 8.8. Solving for fixed cost.

To prove the mathematical accuracy of the above analysis, insert total fixed and the variable cost per unit into the cost formula for March. If it explains the total cost of March, it is mathematically correct. See the proof shown in Figure 8.9.

The high/low method is relatively easy to calculate, however the equation only fits the highest and lowest months because all other interim data were ignored in the computation. Differences caused by using this selective data may be incidental if the differences in monthly activity and costs are not large. The larger the variance, the greater the chance that either the fixed or variable cost component will be disproportionately affected by this method.

Regression Analysis — Mixed Costs

Regression analysis is purported to be the most accurate method of identifying cost behavior patterns. The formula supporting a straight line is

$$Y = a + bX$$

Total Cost	=	Fixed Cost	+	Variable Cost
$9,800	=	$2,150	+	180 units @ $42.50/unit (or $7,650)
$9,800	=	$2,150	+	$7,650

Figure 8.9. Proof: substitution of fixed and variable costs into equation.

Month	Y	X	x	y	xy	y^2
				Difference from Average		
Jan.	$10,500	200	-1,113	-18	20,034	324
Feb.	13,200	260	1,587	42	66,654	1,764
Mar.	9,800	180	-1,813	-38	68,894	1,444
Apr.	11,566	209	- 47	- 9	423	81
May	13,000	243	1,386	25	34,675	625
Totals	$58,066	1,092	-0-	-0-	190,680	4,328
Average	$11,613	218				

$$\text{Variable Rate or } x = \frac{\Sigma xy}{\Sigma y^2} = \frac{190,680}{4,238} = \$44.99$$

$$Y = a + bX$$

$$\$10,500 = a + (200)(\$44.99)$$

$$\text{Fixed cost or } a = \$1,502$$

Where:
X = activity measure
Y = Total cost
a = fixed cost
b = variable rate
n = number of observations

Figure 8.10. Regression analysis example.

with Y the dependent variable and X the independent variable. Applying the rules of least squares to observed activity and cost produces the formula found in Figure 8.10. When the regression or least squares method is used, any month's data can be substituted into the basic formula to solve for variable and fixed costs.

Simple computer software programs can be obtained that will identify fixed cost and variable cost per unit elements by simply inputting activity (the independent variable) and cost data (the dependent variable) for various points in time. There are even some inexpensive pocket calculators that perform the same function.

Activity Base

The activity base assigned to any department should be its nonmonetary method of quantifying work. As such, managers should select the activity unit that best describes and measures work performed. For example, a laboratory could use total number of tests as its work measurement, but there is an inherent error in this selection. Using the number of tests presupposes that every test requires the same use of resources, which is not true. A better labor-activity measurement would be a weighted value derived by multiplying each test by a factor that gives effect to the varying degrees of difficulty and time involved. The name given to this weighted measure is relative value unit (RVU).

Nursing stations must develop a unit of measure that identifies their work performance. Using patient days has the same inherent error built into the base as did the laboratory's unadjusted measure. Managers can develop an RVU for nursing by creating a weighted value to each patient's stay based upon the level of patient acuity. DRG codes can be used to develop RVUs. This weighted value is a better measure of nursing service's work. Nursing labor may serve as the base for determining nursing RVUs in the absence of acuity or other acceptable measures. The simplest patient day can be defined as "1" and other patient days can be valued in relation to the proportionate amount of extra labor hours involved, thus creating the weighted factor.

Once an activity base is identified, the organization must gather and monitor the daily accumulation of data.

Relevant Range

It is important to realize that relationships that exist between costs and a chosen activity base, as previously discussed, are valid only within a relevant range of activity. For example, different cost relationships exist when a department operates at 75% or 85% capacity than when that same department operates at a much lower level of occupancy. Cost relationships change because management adjusts its staffing levels and spends less in an attempt to eliminate certain costs as activity drops. For example, if occupancy drops to 40%, a department that is open 24 hours a day may reduce its shift coverage to 12 or 16 hours, and a nursing unit that is operating at 50% occupancy may be combined with another nursing unit, thereby eliminating the costs associ-

	Amount	Percentage
Revenue	$10,000	100%
Less Variable Costs	$ 6,000	60%
Contribution Margin	$ 4,000	40%
Less Fixed Costs	$ 4,000	40%
Net Income	-0-	-0-

Figure 8.11. Income statement prepared using break-even analysis classifications.

ated with the one unit. As occupancy levels increase, additional beds and eventually entire nursing units may be added. Each of these changes is an example of an institution adjusting its spending patterns to coincide with changes in activity levels that place the institution in a new relevant range. Entering a new range means new cost behavior patterns exist and must be identified. The activity range in which the institution is currently and likely to continue operating is its relevant range. Once the relevant range is determined, managers must identify specific cost/activity relationships associated with it.

BREAK-EVEN ANALYSIS

Managers must know cost behavior patterns to identify the break-even point, the level of activity where revenue exactly equals cost. Break-even analysis is based upon a departmental income statement that separates costs into fixed and variable categories. See Figure 8.11 for a sample income statement prepared using break-even analysis classifications.

Contribution margin is the difference between the average revenue per unit of activity and its variable cost per unit. Using this information, there is a simple formula for calculating the break-even point without using a trial and error approach. These formulae appear in Figure 8.12.

$$\frac{\text{Fixed Cost}}{\text{Contribution Margin Ratio}} = \text{Revenue at break-even}$$

$$\frac{\text{Fixed Cost}}{\text{Contribution Margin/Unit}} = \begin{array}{l} \text{Number of Units of} \\ \text{Activity at Break-even} \end{array}$$

Figure 8.12. Formulae for calculating the break-even point.

For example, if total monthly fixed costs are $3,500, and variable costs are approximately 12 1/2% of revenue, the break-even point is $4,000 of revenue, as calculated in Figure 8.13.

Break-even revenue of $4,000 means that as long as a department earns $4,000 or more from providing services during any month, its revenues should exceed its costs. For every dollar of revenue over $4,000, the department's net income increases by its contribution margin or $0.875.

Armed with this knowledge, and current activity information, managers can predict departmental profits.

Operating Strategies to Increase Net Income

There are three different factors that will affect the department's bottom line or net income. A department can

1. Increase the fee for service.
2. Decrease the cost (either fixed or variable) of providing the service.
3. Increase the volume of services provided.

An approach that includes all three strategies or one that focuses on just one of these strategies may be selected by an individual institution to increase profits.

$$\frac{\text{Fixed Costs}}{\text{Contribution Margin Ratio}} = \frac{\$3,500}{(100\% - 12\ 1/2\%)} = \begin{array}{l} \text{Break-even} \\ \text{Point } \$4,000 \end{array}$$

Figure 8.13. Calculation of break-even point.

Basic Information

Fee charged per procedure	$50
Cost of providing the service	
Salaries (Variable cost/procedure)	$10
Equipment annual depreciation*	
(Fixed Cost)	$1,000
Number of procedures performed annually	40

*Equipment cost is $10,000; expected life is 10 years.

Income Statement Using the Information Basic to the Problem

Revenue (40 @ $50)		$2,000
Salary Expense (40 @ $10)	$ 400	
Depreciation	1,000	(1,400)
Net Income		$ 600
Break-even point		

$$\frac{\text{Fixed Cost}}{\text{Contribution Margin/Unit}} = \frac{\$1,000}{\$50 - \$10} = 25 \text{ procedures}$$

Figure 8.14. Sample information to be applied to increase profits.

Using the information provided in Figure 8.14, the various strategies will be applied to increase profits.

If the fee is increased to $51 per procedure and all other information remains unchanged, the new net income for this procedure becomes $640, an increase of $40 over the base period example (see Figure 8.15).

If the fee remains unchanged, but the institution is able to reduce salary cost to $9.50 per procedure, the organization will report a net income of $620, an increase of $20 over the base period example (see Figure 8.16).

An increase in the number of procedures that are performed during the time period will also increase net income. In this final example, the number of procedures increases by 8, and all other fee and cost data remain unchanged. Results of a volume increase shows an increase in net income of $320 (see Figure 8.17).

Revenue (40 @ $51)		$2,040
Salary Expense (40 @ $10)	$ 400	
Depreciation	1,000	(1,400)
Net Income		$ 640

Break-even point

$$\frac{\text{Fixed Cost}}{\text{Contribution Margin/Unit}} = \frac{\$1,000}{\$51 - \$10} = 24 \text{ procedures}$$

Figure 8.15. Income statement with fee increase of $1 per procedure.

The break-even point remains unchanged at 25 procedures. The distance from break-even point is increased, thus increasing profit by the additional units (8) times the contribution margin of $40 per procedure, or $320.

For institutions that have high fixed costs in their operating statements, the best strategy for increasing net income is to increase activity. In this way, fixed costs can be spread over more procedures, thereby reducing the cost per unit.

Revenue (40 @ $50)		$2,000
Salary Expense (40 @ $9.50)	$ 380	
Depreciation	1,000	(1,380)
Net Income		$ 620

Break-even point

$$\frac{\text{Fixed Cost}}{\text{Contribution Margin/Unit}} = \frac{\$1,000}{\$51 - \$9.50} = 24 \text{ procedures}$$

Figure 8.16. Income statement adjusted for salary reduction of $0.50 per procedure.

Revenue (48 @ $50)		$2,400
Salary Expense (48 @ $10)	$ 480	
Depreciation	1,000	(1,480)
Net Income		$ 920

Figure 8.17. Income statement adjusted for increase in volume.

SUMMARY

Net income is positively affected by fee increases, cost decreases, and/or volume increases. Conversely, net income decreases if fees decrease, costs increase, and/or the volume of services provided decreases.

Readers realize after having read Chapter VII (Economic and Legal Environment of the Health Care Industry) that federal legislation has restricted a hospital's ability to receive payment for increased fees. If Medicare and Medicaid patients represent approximately 40% of the services provided, then 40% of the work performed is being reimbursed at less than full charges.

Most institutions are focussing their attention on cost containment and volume increases as the strategies for increasing profits. Utilization review has effectively reduced inpatient length of stay in most institutions. Therefore, if admissions remain constant or increase slightly over time, the total number of patient days will decrease due to reduced patient stays. Occupancy levels are affected and department capacity may decrease. In response to these changes, health care institutions are emphasizing outpatient services as a means of maintaining their relevant range of activity.

A health care provider's costs within its relevant range of activity are primarily fixed in nature. To lower the cost per patient or case, the best strategy is to increase the volume of procedures, thus providing a broader base over which to spread fixed costs. For that reason, many institutions enter joint venture arrangements and contracts with health maintenance organizations (HMO) and other private insurance carriers to provide services at a fee below that normally charged by the institution. This practice yields added profit as long as the new price is greater than any incremental fixed and variable costs incurred. Increased utilization of the facility causes an increase in profits.

QUESTIONS

1. What is the difference between a fixed cost and a variable cost? Give an example of each.
2. What is a mixed cost? Why is it important to separate the fixed and variable components of a mixed cost?
3. What methods can be used to separate fixed and variable components of a mixed cost?
4. In your opinion, what type of cost behavior pattern would most hospital costs follow?
5. Define break-even. Why is it helpful to know a department's break-even point?
6. What strategies can a department use to increase operating income?

EXERCISES

1. Identify the type of cost behavior (fixed, variable, mixed) that is present in each example. Be prepared to give reasons for your answer.

	May	June	July	August
Level of Activity	**120**	**150**	**140**	**145**
1. Salaries	$1,000	$1,000	$1,000	$1,000
2. Salaries, assistants	1,800	2,250	2,100	2,175
3. Supplies	240	300	280	290
4. Supplies, disposable	290	350	330	340
5. Depreciation	700	700	700	700
6. Other expenses	160	190	180	190

2. Use the information from exercise 1. For those mixed costs, use the high/low method and identify the fixed and variable cost components.

3. Using the information in exercise 1, calculate the total fixed cost that is involved in operating this department.

4. Using the information in exercise 1, calculate the total variable cost per adjusted admission that is involved in operating this department.

5. Using the fixed cost total from exercise 3 and the variable cost per adjusted admission from exercise 4, calculate the expected total costs (both fixed and variable) of the department if it expects to have 130 adjusted admissions next month.

IX

Budgeting

CHAPTER OBJECTIVES

1. Define budgeting.
2. Explain the role that budgeting plays in the management process.
3. Differentiate between short-term and long-term budgets.
4. Identify and explain various budgeting philosophies.
5. Identify and explain various budgeting methodologies.

A budget is a written forecast of the future, quantified in terms of dollar inflows (revenue and/or cash) and dollar outflows (expenses and/or cash). Budgets are prepared as planning tools, used to allocate resources within an entity, and finally used to evaluate operations.

A large entity must divide itself into smaller, more manageable units before preparing a budget. Because hospitals are organized into departments, these departments become the basis for budgeting. Departments may be referred to as revenue-producing or nonrevenue-producing cost centers. This depends on whether the unit provides service and bills the ultimate consumer. Some nonrevenue-producing cost centers that generate no revenue, only costs, are patient accounts, maintenance, laundry, and housekeeping.

Departments that generate revenue as well as costs (revenue centers or revenue-producing cost centers) include laboratory, radiology, surgery, and other ancillary departments. In general, nursing stations, plus labor, delivery and operating rooms, are revenue centers with their revenue credited to nursing service.

BUDGETING AS A TOOL ————————————————

A budget is a management tool that enables an entity to

1. Plan for future operations.
2. Direct daily operations.
3. Control expenditures.
4. Evaluate each component's ability to operate efficiently and effectively in the marketplace.

These four functions define the basic tasks that all managers must perform.

Planning

Planning is a difficult task for most managers because it takes them out of an active role and forces them to study what has been and is continuing to happen to and within their departments. The ultimate goal of planning is to project future demand for services. This task is especially difficult if technology keeps changing the nature of the services provided. Planning is one of the most important management functions because it provides managers with an intuitive knowledge of the individual unit's needs, challenges, and alternatives. Managers must be sensitive to resource needs and assess alternative courses of action so that they can anticipate problems before they materialize. For instance, managers may schedule employee vacations during anticipated slack times; order inventory in advance of peak utilization periods; or shift nursing personnel and/or patients, if possible, to better match resources and needs. Advance planning is necessary for implementing new medical procedures, especially when those procedures require in-service training and additional supplies and equipment.

Directing and Organizing

To direct and organize, managers must know what assets are available. A budget, prepared at the beginning of each year, serves as a formal request for departmental resources. Department managers prepare budget requests and submit them to administration. All departments submit similar requests for asset allocations. Because hospital resources are limited, not all requests can be honored, and many times the final budget is the result of negotiations and compromises made by both administration and hospital managers.

Once accepted by both parties, a budget serves as a written statement of future resource allocations. These resource allocations are conditional upon the realization of anticipated demand. First-line managers can use their budget as a tool to order and charge resources to their department. Budgeting records also provide managers with a measure of actual usage against what was expected.

Controlling

By comparing actual activity levels, revenue, and expenses to their budgeted counterparts for the same time period, managers can review and investigate major differences as they arise. Management by exception helps managers focus on major differences only.

Encoding errors occur when expenses charged to one department were incurred somewhere else, and they may be the source of differences. A review of budget versus actual costs provides internal control and helps managers identify such errors. They can then be corrected and separated from departmental financial information, allowing only actual differences to surface.

Areas of concern can be identified early and alternative courses of action assessed. Advance warning gives managers the lead time needed to gather information on alternatives and then select that course of action best suited for the department and the institution.

Evaluating Performance

Evaluation uses hindsight to assess an organization's ability to operate profitably within its environment. This process reviews the entire organization by concentrating on its major activities and the work performed by individual departments. Evaluation is performed at every level of management, beginning with department managers and continuing to the chief executive officer.

If a unit is operating efficiently, management may decide to maintain the status quo. If activity levels are greater than anticipated, management may review operations to determine whether this trend is a temporary or permanent change. A decrease in activity requires similar analysis. If the change is considered temporary, temporary budget additions or cutbacks may be initiated. Where possible, employee hours may be adjusted. Part-time employees may be used to meet increased demand as activity rises. If activity decreases, employee positions vacated through normal attrition may be left unfilled or canceled entirely. New programs may be initiated earlier than planned or postponed indefinitely.

Permanent changes in activity levels require permanent changes in the level of spending. If a change in service level occurs, nurse/patient ratios may be adjusted, the mix of nurses used (degreed versus nondegreed) may be altered, or ancillary department response time for posting procedure results may be changed.

Departmental changes must be viewed in total to determine if one department's increased activity is offset by another's decrease, or whether that department's change is indicative of a new trend or change in the region's demand for health care.

BUDGETING PHILOSOPHIES ——————————

Top-down Philosophy

Budgets may be prepared under one of two philosophies. Budgets may be prepared by top administration and passed down to each department. This is the top-down philosophy. This budgeting philosophy is often very effectual in anticipating demand for services. It also takes less time to prepare this type of budget, and spares first-line managers the headaches associated with budgeting. Budgets prepared in this manner will give first-line managers information regarding available departmental resources. However, top-down budgets lose some of their efficacy as a tool for directing and controlling operations.

Because their input was not incorporated, first-line managers may not accept the budget as a realistic assessment of how their unit should perform. In many instances, the budget may be viewed as the administration's budget and personal incentives to meet to budget projections may not exist. Top-down philosophy may lead administration and first-line managers to adversarial positions, or first-line managers may cut their unit's costs to remain within budget, when those added costs may have been needed to service above-budget activity. Strict adherence to the budget may later prove detrimental to the entity. For example, to reduce costs, managers may refuse preventive maintenance or delay ordering necessary supplies. Later equipment failures and inventory shortages may prove more costly than initial expenditures. Administration and department managers must cooperate to alleviate some of these problems.

Bottom-up Philosophy

An alternative budgeting philosophy, or bottom-up approach, involves active participation from all levels of management during the entire budgeting process. Department managers begin this process by planning or forecasting for the next year, converting this plan into budgeted revenues and expenses. Proposed budgets are then given to administration for discussion, negotiation, and approval. The budget becomes the joint product of all levels of management.

Besides instilling a sense of cooperation within the organization, the bottom-up budgeting philosophy gives department managers added incentive to make their budget work. This philosophy also taps a major source of information because first-line managers know the operating intricacies of their units better than anyone else. By enlisting their cooperation, hospitals benefit from their added knowledge and insight. In addition, managers are sensitized to the impact that their daily decisions have on operations and profitability.

Actual Practice

Actual organizational budgeting philosophies generally fall somewhere between these two extremes. Top administration generally assists department managers by projecting activity levels for revenue centers. Administration may even establish fee schedules for room rates, tests, and procedures. Finance personnel often calculate total revenue by extending and totalling amounts. Other departments such as personnel and purchasing offer their expertise by predicting changes that managers can expect in manpower and supply costs. Managers then use all this information to prepare their actual budgets.

Negotiations still occur between administration and individual departments regarding the manner in which activity levels are converted to dollar values, especially because available resources are limited. Once all parties agree, budgets become the management tool that they were intended to be.

BUDGET TIME FRAMES ————————————————

Budgets are prepared for two different time periods. Short-range budgets are prepared for one year, while long-range budgets are prepared for anywhere from five to ten years.

Short-range Budgets

Short-range budgets focus on planning for the immediate, succeeding year. Since this time period is close at hand, it is necessary to have explicit detailed cost and revenue projections. Short-range budgets are generally prepared by department managers and submitted to administration (assuming the bottom-up philosophy is adopted). They include forecasted revenue and expense for each unit. Other details may be highlighted, such as revenue by patient classification, inpatient or outpatient, and expense by account classification. Short-range budgets may be prepared for the entire next year, with monthly budgets derived by dividing the total by twelve. Another option is that managers may be permitted to assign cost and revenue to specific months in which they are expected to occur.

Long-range Budgets

Long-range budgets forecast operations for many years into the future. The length of time depends on administration's views of the economy, its environment, and the stability of each. Because this budget is projected much further into the future, there is more room for change over time. For this reason, long-range budgets are not prepared in detail. This budget process must analyze the hospital's economic environment and identify present and expected changes in health care delivery systems. It also identifies new areas of specialty services, as well as geographic locations where service demands may surface. Long-range budgets also identify space and facility needs and, with that, construction and financing requirements.

Long-range budgets are generally prepared by a long-range planning committee of the hospital with input from department heads, medical staff, and area experts. Before the long-range budgeting process can begin, organizational goals, such as the geographic region to be served and the nature and extent of the services to be provided, must be identified and agreed upon.

With these goals in mind, a hospital can assess needed resources and when these needs will arise. Reassessment of organizational goals and industry environment are intricate parts of this long-range budgeting process. Administration may need to enlist the forecasting abilities of such experts as economists, lawyers, legislators, bankers, financial planners, and engineers.

New data can be incorporated into long-range projections as it becomes available. For example, expansion of institutional goals to offer a full spectrum of health care services could lead to the purchase of land as a future site for a nursing home or satellite unit. If internal studies and area experts agree that there is sufficient need to justify this endeavor, an institution could begin seeking approval from area planning councils and local zoning boards. A hospital might seek to purchase land and construct its own facility, or shop around for an existing facility. There would be ample time to review financing needs and any legal issues associated with off-site operations.

Long-range plans must be converted into long-range budgets that identify revenues, expenses, cash receipts, and cash disbursements for all years covered by the budget. These budgets are not prepared in detail, and generally include projected building and equipment expenditures. They identify operating resources that will be needed to start new programs or open new units. Long-range budgets manage by exception and only address changes, programs, or services that will be initiated in the future or existing programs that may be changed or canceled.

At some point in time, long-range budgets overlap short-range budgets. As time approaches for a new nursing home or satellite unit to open, detailed departmental budgets must be prepared. Personnel and supply needs are converted into expected cost data by category of expense, and demand is converted to budgeted revenue. Planning remains the major benefit of long-range budgeting.

Long-range budgeting also forces top management to choose between alternatives before any resources are committed. An institution will be able to capitalize on changes as opportunities arise because mechanisms for making changes are already in place.

OPERATING VERSUS CAPITAL BUDGETS _____

In addition to dealing with various time frames, an organization must deal with budgeting for different types of resources. Operating budgets deal with planning for ongoing operations. Capital budgeting concerns itself with planning for fixed asset acquisitions and disposals. In general, operating and capital budgets follow the short-term/long-term budget dichotomy.

Operating Budgets

Operating budgets cover daily activities and are usually prepared for short terms, whereas long-range budgets cover facility acquisitions and financing requirements needed to support entity changes. There is some overlap of planning activities as long-range plans enter the short-term time period. The results of operations are reflected in individual departmental income statements and collectively in an entity's income statement. Operating budgets are projected income statements for next year. They include estimates of future activity converted into revenue and expenses.

Capital Budgets

Capital budgets address anticipated purchases of property, plant, and equipment only, fixed assets that are reflected in balance sheet accounts. Departmental managers may be required to complete and submit fixed asset requisitions. These capital expenditures will only cross their income statements as depreciation expenses. Most organizations reflect depreciation as a one-line expense category on their income statement and do not charge it directly to individual departments. Therefore, managers do not see the increased expense resulting from capital acquisitions.

BUDGETING APPROACHES ———————————————

Line-item Budgeting

Projections of future costs are often based upon past experience. An entity's approach to budgeting depends upon which, if any, historical costs are accepted as foundation for future cost predictions. Many institutions use the prior year's actual costs as the starting point for preparing budgets for subsequent years. Line-item budgeting uses last year's actual costs and revenue and adjusts them for expected changes in activity levels and prices.

Zero-based Budgeting

Zero-based budgeting starts by accepting none of last year's actual costs. Managers must justify every budget dollar. First, managers predict activity levels. They then project labor and supplies needed to perform the anticipated work. During this process, managers must verify these needs by showing detailed resource requirements by units of work. Total budgets are calculated by multiplying individual resource needs by number of work units expected to be performed.

Program Budgeting

A third approach to budgeting exists, although it is rarely used by existing departments. Program budgeting works best when departments have been given seed money to accomplish a specific task. In this situation, managers are given the total amount that can be spent. No other constraints are placed on how monies are to be used. Managers may hire new employees, subcontract labor requirements, purchase supplies, or rent equipment, as long as the task is accomplished within the budget limits.

ADVANTAGES AND DISADVANTAGES OF BUDGETING APPROACHES _____

Ease of Budget Preparation

Of the three alternatives (line-item, zero-based, and program), line-item budgeting is the easiest to prepare and therefore takes the least time and effort. Historical costs are accepted as the starting point. Budgets are prepared by incorporating the effects of expected activity and resource price changes into last year's data.

Program budgeting is more difficult than line-item budgeting because managers must formulate a spending plan where none existed. Even though no detailed restrictions are placed upon funds, managers should project expense categories. This approach involves more preparation time and effort.

Zero-based budgeting is the most difficult and time-consuming approach because managers must support and justify every budget dollar. Time and motion studies may be necessary. Managers may also use outside data gathered by independent studies.

Cost Containment

Line-item budgeting will perpetuate waste if it exists within the base period. For example, if a nursing unit is overstaffed initially, this budgeting approach will not identify that this problem exists. It will add additional costs for increased activity and price changes.

Program budgeting uses activity and dollar constraints as spending limitations. Waste may occur but it will not necessarily be perpetuated because of the limited nature of the assignment.

Zero-based budgeting is designed to eliminate waste. Elimination of waste and improper use of hospital resources is its primary purpose.

In general, line-item budgeting is utilized by most health care institutions. Occasionally, when the administration believes that resources are not being utilized properly, it may require specific departments to use an alternative budgeting approach. The one usually recommended is zero-based budgeting.

Perfect versus Normal Utilization of Resources

A budget should estimate expected costs and revenues, knowing full well that human beings comprise the hospital community. Humans are unable to give 100% of their energies all the time. There will be times when employees become ill and are unable to work at peak performance, if at all. Supplies will be spilled and forms redone. These types of occurrences result in real world operations. Some imperfection is inevitable because of the human element.

A budget should allow for normal human imperfections. The key becomes including only a minimal level of inefficiency. For a budget to serve as an evaluation tool, it must identify what are reasonable future costs and revenue expectations. Budgets prepared under assumptions of perfect resource utilization will always fall short of realization. Differences or variances will always occur. It will be difficult to separate improper resource utilization from normal human inefficiency. Also, managers become frustrated because even their best efforts will not succeed in eliminating variances. Therefore, budgets should be prepared under assumptions of normal behavior. Then, any differences between actual and budgeted costs will have an explanation.

SUMMARY

The budget forecasts the future of an organization in terms of dollar inflows and outflows. It is a management tool that enables an entity to plan for future operations, to direct daily operations, to control expenditures, and to evaluate each component's ability to operate efficiently and effectively in the market place.

Budgets are prepared under either the top-down (top administration prepares it and passes it down to each department) or bottom-up (involves all levels of management in preparation) philosophy. Actual budgeting generally falls somewhere in between these two philosophies.

Budgets can be prepared for either the short range (in the next year) or long range (for anywhere from five to ten years). Short-range budgets are very explicit and detailed, whereas long-range budgets are not prepared in detail. A hospital's goals define which type of budget should be used.

There are two different budgets that deal with different types of resources: operating and capital budgets. Operating budgets, which are usually prepared for short terms, help plan for ongoing operations. Capital budgets deal with planning for fixed asset acquisitions and disposals, which are long-range projects. There is some overlap of the two types of budgets.

Budgeting can be approached in three ways. Line-item budgeting, which uses the previous year's actual costs and revenue as a base, is the easiest approach. Zero-based budgeting starts from scratch and managers must justify every budget dollar. Program budgeting takes place when managers are given the total amount that can be spent and no constraints are placed on spending. Zero-based budgeting is the most difficult and time-consuming budgeting approach that an entity can take. But, when cost containment is the focal point, zero-based budgeting has the greatest tendency to eliminate unnecessary costs.

QUESTIONS ───────────────────────────────

1. Define budgeting.
2. What function does budgeting serve? Explain your answer.
3. What is the difference between short-term and long-term budgets? Who is responsible for each and how detailed does each become?
4. What is a budgeting philosophy?
5. How does an entity's budgeting philosophy affect the division of duties; the department's level of responsibility for achieving its estimates; the time that it takes to prepare the budget; and the involvement of the various levels of management?
6. Give the various approaches that an entity may take in preparing its budget. Give the advantages and disadvantages of each approach.

X

Budgeting Requirements

CHAPTER OBJECTIVES

1. Identify specific departmental information that is needed for budgeting.
2. Identify questions that managers should ask before the budgeting process can begin.

The costs charged to individual departments and the method of charging costs vary among hospitals. Before the budgeting process can begin, managers must be certain that they know exactly which costs are being charged to their department, and which mechanisms trigger charges. It is essential that managers know how their specific institution handles each of the following items.

Salaries Paid for Nonworked Hours

A full-time employee is paid for approximately 2,080 hours during a year (40 hours each week for 52 weeks). For this reason, 2,080 hours of work is referred to as one full-time equivalent (FTE) employee. Not all of the paid hours represent work hours because all institutions have vacation plans that cover permanent full-time and some, if not all, permanent part-time employees. They also have other fringe benefits such as sick leave and in-service education. Institutions vary in their choice of which cost center receives these paid, nonworked hours. Some institutions charge the home department for vacation, sick, holiday, and other comparable items, while others charge nonworked, paid time to the Personnel or Human Resources cost center. Still others establish and charge a separate cost center called Employee Fringe Benefits. In the first instance, the home department must include the vacation, sick, and other nonworked hours and costs in its budget. In the second and third examples, the department ignores these items and reduces salary expense by their cost.

Employee Replacement

After managers determine the base personnel costs charged to their department, they must review hospital policy for replacing absent employees with temporary workers. Many hospitals use nursing pools or floats (a department of permanently employed nurses who move from department to department on an "as needed" basis) to cover temporary personnel shortages. It is important to know where these hours are charged.

Most hospitals charge replacement time directly to the using department, making that department manager responsible for supervising the work and signing time cards. However, there are some hospitals that charge these hours and costs to a separate home department called Pools and Floats, or to Nursing Administration itself.

The examples shown in Figures 10.1–10.3 depict the impact that each alternative has on the departmental personnel hours. The department in question is staffed by one full-time employee (FTE) and that employee is entitled to the following benefits: 1) 2 weeks vacation (80 hours), 2) 7 holidays (56 hours), and 3) 12 days of sick leave of which the employee is expected to use 5 (40 hours). The employee's base pay is $10.00 per hour.

To adjust this example for a specific department, select the example that explains salary expense and adjust the vacation and sick hours to the average taken by employees. Then multiply total hours for the adjusted example by the number of full-time equivalent employees that are assigned to the department. The product will be total budgeted salary expense.

Supply Costs

Several mechanisms may be used to charge supply costs to departments. An inventory cart system charges departments as inventory levels are replenished. Supply charges also may result from ordering and receiving supplies directly from outside vendors. In the first instance, the expense is charged to the department at regular intervals, probably

Base hours of full-time employee	2,080
Replacement time for vacation	80
Replacement time for 7 holidays	56
Replacement time for sick leave	40
Total hours charged to the department	2,256
Total cost charged to department	
(2,256 hours @ $10 per hours)	$22,560

Figure 10.1. Vacation time, sick leave, and replacement time are charged to the department.

Base hours of employee	2,080
Less vacation, holiday, and sick hours charged to Fringe Benefits	(176)
Add replacement time charged to the department	176
Total hours charged to the department	2,080
Total cost charged to the department	
(2,080 hours @ $10 per hour)	$20,800

Figure 10.2. Vacation, holiday, and sick pay is charged to a fringe benefit account that is not a cost to the department. Replacement time is charged to the department.

Base hours of employee	2,080
Less vacation, holiday, and sick hours charged Fringe Benefit account	(176)
Total hours charged to the department	1,904
Total cost charged to the department	
(1,904 hours @ $10 per hour)	$19,040

Figure 10.3. Vacation, holiday, and sick pay is charged to the fringe benefit account, not to the department. Replacement time is charged to Nursing Administration.

at weekly or biweekly intervals. Charging supplies using the second method is not as predictable because goods must be received and their invoices processed before charges appear on the departmental financial statements. The time period between these two occurrences often involves several days, weeks, or even months.

Departmental Information That Must Be Reviewed and Gathered

Before budgeting, managers must gather all cost and activity information associated with the current year. The best scenario has managers receiving monthly departmental financial statements that give each period's actual costs, budgeted costs, and actual and budgeted activity. It is helpful if this statement also gives year-to-date information for costs and activity. Managers must accumulate this information in situations where it is not provided on periodic reports.

Cost and revenue should go hand in hand. The revenue generated by providing services or selling goods should be credited to the department that carries its cost. Occasionally, revenue and costs are inadvertently separated. Managers should ascertain that all revenue earned by their departments is reported within their departmental statements.

Regardless of form, periodic financial reports must be scrutinized when received and discrepancies should be investigated immediately. Notations can be made of unique occurrences, such as use of overtime to staff the unit during a flu epidemic or the extra time and staff involved in the training of new hires, as they happen. Postponing the review until later dates robs managers of causal information, often resulting in added time spent on reconstructions. This may also lead to improper conclusions. Other reports support financial statement charges. There should be internal payroll schedules and reports supporting departmental hours and salaries expense by pay period. Again, a current review of all reports will catch errors in assigning and charging personnel time. Depending upon the individual institution, other reports of items such as supplies and expense items may also be made available as detail support.

The activity base selected as the best unit for identifying work performed and explaining cost changes from period to period should be analyzed to see if it is still the best one available. Additional research in work measurement and added expertise may yield new and better work measures.

Financial reports must be analyzed and cost behavior patterns related to activity levels identified. These will form the basis for making future predictions.

If managers forecast activity levels, then trends for the last year should be reviewed. Generally, the administration accumulates and analyzes past data and predicts future activity levels that are then forwarded to respective departments.

ALLOCATING THE ANNUAL BUDGET TO THE MONTHS OF THE YEAR

Most managers project the total budget for the next operating year, rather than budgeting by month and summing the costs. If this is the case, several options are available for assigning specific costs to specific months of the year (see Figure 10.4). While their availability will depend on computer capabilities, the method used will directly affect projected monthly costs and revenue.

Division by Twelve

A common approach to preparing monthly budgets is to take total annual costs and divide them by twelve. This method is simple, but it builds inherent month-end variances into the actual revenue cost versus budget analysis revenue cost because months are not alike in the number of days, nor in the level of activity expected.

Proportional Allocation Based upon Days of Year

A second alternative is to allocate costs to each month in direct proportion to their share of the year's time. While this method allows for the differences that exist in the actual number of days per month, it does not provide for any seasonal differences. For example, December is typically a low-revenue month because there are fewer inpatients admitted during the holiday season. The variable expenses that are associated with inpatient stays should be lower during this month. However, since December is a month with 31 days, it would be allocated the same supply expense as January and July.

Budget for Month is 1/12 of Year

19__ Budgeted Expense	JAN	FEB	MAR	APR	MAY	JUN	JUL	AUG	SEP	OCT	NOV	DEC
Salary $24,000	$2,000	$2,000	$2,000	$2,000	$2,000	$2,000	$2,000	$2,000	$2,000	$2,000	$2,000	$2,000
Supplies $6,000	500	500	500	500	500	500	500	500	500	500	500	500
Expense $2,400	200	200	200	200	200	200	200	200	200	200	200	200

Budget for Month Based on Month's Days

	JAN	FEB	MAR	APR	MAY	JUN	JUL	AUG	SEP	OCT	NOV	DEC
Salary $24,000	$2,038	$1,841	$2,038	$1,972	$2,038	$1,972	$2,038	$2,038	$1,972	$2,038	$1,972	$2,038
Supplies $6,000	509	460	509	493	509	493	509	509	493	509	493	509
Expense $2,400	204	184	204	197	204	197	204	204	197	204	197	204

Budget for Month Based on Prior Actual Cost As Percent of Last Year's Total Expense

	JAN	FEB	MAR	APR	MAY	JUN	JUL	AUG	SEP	OCT	NOV	DEC
$30,000	$2,400	$2,100	$2,100	$3,000	$2,400	$3,300	$2,400	$3,000	$2,400	$1,800	$2,100	$3,000
Percent of Total	8%	7%	7%	10%	8%	11%	8%	10%	8%	6%	7%	10%

19__ Budget Expense

	JAN	FEB	MAR	APR	MAY	JUN	JUL	AUG	SEP	OCT	NOV	DEC
Salary $24,000	$1,920	$1,680	$1,680	$2,400	$1,920	$2,640	$1,920	$2,400	$1,920	$1,440	$1,680	$2,400
Supplies $6,000	480	420	420	600	480	660	480	600	480	360	420	600
Expense $2,400	192	168	168	240	192	264	192	240	192	144	168	240

Proportional Allocation Based upon Prior Year's Costs

A third method of spreading the total budget allocates amounts to each month at the same rate that last year's costs were incurred. In this manner, seasonal trends or patterns that repeat themselves are included in the budget, and it automatically adjusts for the differences between the number of days in each month.

The comparison of actual and budgeted costs is an important tool that helps managers keep departments on target and within their budget. Therefore, the better the budget estimates, the greater the ability to use budgets to evaluate and control costs.

Budget flexibility is important. There may be instances when a department knows that a specific expense, such as in-service education, will occur within a specific month. It would be helpful if the budget allocation method allowed for these special instances and provided a means to insert specific costs into specific months.

SUMMARY

Before preparing next year's budget, managers must be aware of current activity and cost levels and know what costs are charged to their department. Nonworked hours, including vacation, sick, and replacement hours, can affect a specific unit's budget in different ways.

There are several options for assigning specific costs to specific months of the year: total annual costs can be divided by twelve; costs can then be allocated to each month in proportion to their share of the year's time; or amounts can be allocated to each month at the same rate as last year's costs were incurred.

A review of prior periods' financial reports and knowledge of how that information is generated will furnish managers increased understanding of their unit's personnel and supply needs.

QUESTIONS

1. Why is it important to know where employee benefit hours are charged?
2. What alternatives can be used for charging employee benefit hours?

3. Give examples of when replacing employees will affect a unit's budgetary computations.
4. How can supply charges differ depending upon the mechanism used for expensing goods? How will this affect a specific unit?
5. What are the methods that an individual institution may use to allocate annual budget amounts to specific months? How can the method used affect a specific department's interpretation of its budget to actual costs for that period?

XI

Exercises in Preparing the Budget

CHAPTER OBJECTIVES

1. Identify information necessary for preparing the budget.
2. Suggest a methodology to be used for preparing budgets.
3. Relate cost/activity relationships to specific budgeting problems.

Budgeting is a planning exercise and, before beginning, managers need to gather the following data.

1. Previous monthly and quarterly financial statements, including actual cost and activity information for the current year
2. A projection of next year's level of activity
3. Employee work-hour information, including employee hours charged to the unit in the past and the approved number of employees assigned to the department
4. Projections of cost increases for salaries (from personnel or human resources department) as well as projections of cost increases for supplies and other expenses (from purchasing or obtained directly from vendors)
5. Any cost constraints placed upon the budget by administration

This exercise involves preparing a budget of 6 West, a 30-bed medical unit. Year-to-date costs for the nursing unit are provided in Figure 11.1.

After this data has been assembled, managers review next year's activity projections. This exercise does not contain a change in the

---

Activity: Adjusted Patient Days   8,450

Actual Cost Information

Salaries, head nurse	$ 38,500
Salaries, nursing	420,000
Salaries, other	75,000
Supplies, disposable	25,350
Supplies, medical	22,000
Supplies, office	4,000
Other expense	13,000
Total	$597,850

Actual worked hours:
    Head nurse   3,208 hours @ average pay of $12.00 per hour
    Nursing   46,667 hours @ average pay of $9.00 per hour
    Technician 12,500 hours @ average pay of $6.00 per hour

Figure 11.1. Year-to-date costs for the nursing unit.

level of service. The only expected changes are due to the following expected cost increases.

1. Salary costs are expected to increase by 3%.
2. Supply costs and other expenses are expected to increase by 4%.
3. Administration expects the level of activity to remain the same.

The following pay policies are in effect for this institution: 1) vacation and sick time are charged to the fringe benefit account that is included in personnel's budget, and 2) replacement help is used and charged to the unit. Figure 11.2 shows the budget calculated under the given budget assumptions.

Figure 11.3 uses the information contained in the original budget and includes an expected increase in activity level. This exercise will use the basic information contained in 6 West and include an increase in activity to 9,295 adjusted patient days for next year. This represents an increase of 10% over current year statistics.

	Actual Cost Current Year	$ Increase in Costs	Budget Next Year
Salaries, head nurse	$38,500	1,155*	39,655
Salaries, nursing	420,000	12,600*	432,600
Salaries, other	75,000	2,250*	77,250
Supplies, disposable	25,350	1,014**	26,364
Supplies, medical	22,000	880**	22,880
Supplies, other	4,000	160**	4,160
Other expense	13,000	520**	13,520
Total	$ 597,850	$18,579	$616,429

* Represents an increase of 3% on current-year cost.
** Represents an increase of 4% of current-year cost.

Figure 11.2. The budget calculated under given budget assumptions.

Using the high/low method of cost identification, the unit's manager determines the cost behavior patterns that follow, as shown in Figure 11.4.

	(A) Fixed Cost	(B) Variable Cost*	(C) Total (A+B)	(D) Price Increase **	(E) Total (C+D)
Salaries, head nurse	$ 38,500	–	$ 38,500	$ 1,155	$ 39,655
Salaries, nursing	251,000	$185,900	436,900	13,107	450,007
Salaries, other	66,550	9,295	75,845	2,275	78,120
Supplies, disposable	–	27,885	27,885	1,115	29,000
Supplies, medical	300	24,167	24,467	979	25,446
Supplies other	2,310	1,859	4,169	167	4,336
Other expense	13,000	–	13,000	520	13,520
Total	$371,660	$249,106	$620,766	$19,318	$640,084

* The variable cost per unit as given in Figure 11.4 was multiplied by the budgeted patient activity of 9,295 units.
**The price increase is calculated by multiplying the total in column "C" by 3% when the cost category is salaries, and 4% when the cost category is supplies or other.

Figure 11.3. Resulting budget calculations.

Cost Category	Fixed Cost	Variable Cost/per Activity Unit
Salary, head nurse	$ 38,500	-0-
Salary, nursing	251,000	$20/unit
Salary, other	66,550	$ 1/unit
Supplies, disposable	-0-	$ 3/unit
Supplies, medical	300	$2.60/unit
Supplies, other	2,310	$0.20/unit
Other expense	13,000	-0-

Figure 11.4. Cost behavior patterns that follow.

EXERCISES

1. An analysis of the monthly costs that were charged to nursing unit 5 West revealed the following patterns:

Salaries	$1,000	+$2/adjusted patient admission
Supplies	-0-	0.50/adjusted patient admission
Other	100	-0-

Administration expects adjusted patient admissions to be 200 for the month. What would be the budgeted expenses for that level of activity?

2. If, in addition to the expected activity level of 200 adjusted patient admissions for next month, Personnel predicted an average increase in salaries of 1% and Purchasing predicted an average increase in supplies and other expense items of 5%, what would be the budgeted expenses for next month?

3. Using the cost behavior patterns given in Figure 11.4, prepare the next year's budget for this nursing unit, assuming that the activity level is expected to drop to 8,000 units.

4. What staffing difficulties will be present if there are wide fluctuations in activity from month to month, and from year to year? What steps might a hospital take to alleviate some of these problems?

5. Will the difficulties associated with staffing for the wide range of activities have the same affect on supplies and other expense? Explain.

XII

The Evaluation Process

CHAPTER OBJECTIVES

1. Give a methodology for isolating differences between actual and budgeted amounts.
2. Identify control methods that can be used to bring costs in line with budget projections.

For added control, departmental financial reports providing actual and budgeted revenue and expense should be prepared and distributed monthly. Reporting format will differ among institutions; year-to-date actual and budget information may be reported, as well as budgeted versus actual activity data. If year-to-date financial information and activity data are missing, managers will have to maintain and accumulate this information on their own.

A variance exists when actual amounts differ from those budgeted. Reasons behind variances may result from several factors, such as actual operations being at a different activity level than expected. A comparison of actual and budgeted levels of activity will disclose this information. If the difference in the activity level is great, budget projections for that month will not provide a valid comparison for actual costs. Figure 12.1 gives an example of actual-versus-budget comparison at month's-end.

It is unfair to compare costs associated with one operating level to the budget of another level. Budget information can and should be adjusted. The adjustment will not occur within the financial statement itself. Using data collected from departmental operations, managers can prepare a new, flexible budget to serve as a valid comparison for actual period costs.

In Figure 12.1, this department appears to have operated satisfactorily because actual costs are less than what was budgeted. For that

	Actual	**Budget**	**Variance***
Salaries	$25,000	$26,100	($ 1,100)
Supplies	800	900	(100)
Other	855	900	(45)
Total	$26,655	$27,900	($ 1,245)
Patient Activity	1,000	1,200	(200)

*( ) indicate that actual costs are less than budget.

Figure 12.1.   Actual-versus-budget comparison.

reason, managers might not check into these variances because they are favorable. A major difference between actual and budgeted activity levels necessitates further analysis and a budget must be prepared for the 1,000 activity level. A flexible budget converts a standard budget prepared for one activity level to one based on actual activity.

To begin this process, managers must know what cost/volume behavior patterns exist for this department. Cost/volume behaviors for the previous department are repeated in Figure 12.2. Using this additional information, managers can prepare a flexible budget for the 1,000-unit level of activity, as shown in Figure 12.3.

This flexible budget offers a fair comparison for the month's actual costs, and it isolates variances, which provides managers with ammunition needed for seeking the reasons behind the variances. Managers should maintain a diary and make notations on staffing changes and their reasons, as well as changes in supply usage. Any information that can help explain month-end variances should be kept. Remember that a hospital's method of allocating its annual budget amounts to the various months may influence variances.

Managers should minimize their time and maximize their effort and investigate the largest, relative variances first. They should know where to look for details behind their department's costs. If salaries generated a variance, payroll reports should be scrutinized; supply cost variances mean reviewing requisitions, invoices, and central store charges. It is always possible that a cost is charged to the wrong de-

Salaries	Mixed cost	$14,100 + $10/unit of activity
Supplies	Variable Cost	$ 7.50/unit of activity
Other	Fixed	$900

Figure 12.2. Cost/volume behaviors for department in Figure 12.1.

	Budget 1,000 Units	Actual 1,000 Units	Variance*
Salaries	$25,100	$25,000	($ 100)
Supplies	750	800	50
Other	900	855	(45)
Total	$26,750	$27,655	$ (95)

* ( ) indicate that actual costs are less than budgeted costs.

Figure 12.3. Flexible budget for 1,000 units.

partment. Therefore, details of costs should be reviewed to identify major differences.

If actual data is correct and unfavorable variances result, managers must direct their attention to the trouble areas. The discussion should be brought to the department to see if reasons for differences can be isolated and corrected.

SUMMARY

Entities do not often achieve their budgeted level of activity. In those instances where the activity level is missed, budget-versus-actual comparisons are invalid. Managers can make a meaningful comparison by preparing a flexible budget using cost behavior patterns identified in previous chapters and applying them to the current activity level. Using a flexible budget for comparison, managers can isolate variances, identify areas that need to be evaluated, and explain why costs are different than expected.

QUESTIONS

1. Explain why budget-to-actual analysis may be distorted and how the variance may not represent an accurate reflection of what happened during the period.
2. What tool can the manager use to bring budget and actual into a realistic basis for comparison?
3. What is a flexible budget?
4. Will the results of a comparison of budget to actual vary greatly from month to month if activity does not vary between budget and actual?
5. Will a flexible budget for a unit change from period to period if activity changes and the costs are considered to be fixed?
6. What impact does the method that the hospital uses to spread the budget to the months have upon budget-to-actual comparisons for a period?

EXERCISES

1. Given below is the budget information for this nursing unit at the 100-unit level of activity. Prepare a flexible budget for the 80- and 120-unit levels of activity. You may assume that these activities are within the relevant range.

Salaries, Head Nurse (fixed)	$ 2,000
Salaries, Nursing (variable)	10,000
Supplies (variable)	1,000
Other (fixed)	500
Total	$13,500

2. Would your answer to #1 have changed if 80 units was outside the relevant range?

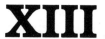

XIII

Cost Allocations

Hospital Organization

Every hospital has revenue-producing departments and nonrevenue-producing or service departments. While revenue-producing departments provide direct patient services and charge fees for these services, nonrevenue-producing departments serve and maintain the revenue producers. Overhead is the name given to costs incurred to keep the hospital operating. This does not include direct materials and direct labor of revenue-producing departments. All costs, both direct and indirect, of nonrevenue-producing departments are general overhead. Fees for service must cover all of the costs of providing the service to enable the hospital to stay in business.

Service or Nonrevenue-producing Departments

There are many nonrevenue-producing departments within a hospital. Their exact number will vary with an institution's size and specialty.

Service or nonrevenue-producing departments include, but are not limited to, hospital administration, maintenance, plant operation, laundry, and housekeeping. To determine a fee for service, it becomes necessary to identify the total cost of providing patient services; therefore, overhead costs associated with service departments must be systematically allocated to revenue-producing departments. How to achieve this goal is the question.

Service department costs may not be charged directly to revenue-producing departments for a number of reasons. First, direct charges would reduce the service department's costs and impede accountability of service department managers. Secondly, internal reports would be difficult to understand. Finally, Medicare cost reporting (HIM—15) forbids the practice of direct charging. Consequently, allocation has been chosen as the process of assigning costs.

Allocation of Nonrevenue-producing Departments

Allocation is accomplished outside of daily accounting transactions. Department costs are charged directly to each department, establishing it as a cost center. Each service department defines its work and identifies a realistic and logical activity base for allocating its costs. For example, maintenance might logically select square footage as their base for allocating cost because maintenance is responsible for the institution's upkeep, and each square foot of space shares equally in the cost of maintenance. All that is needed for allocation is a measurement of hospital square footage by department.

Another allocation base could have been chosen. Maintenance costs could be allocated on the basis of maintenance personnel's assigned time, a statistic that requires more time and effort to accumulate. Using this base, maintenance accumulates worked hours as recorded on work orders. Whereas square footage is a relatively constant statistic, worked hours will change from period to period, requiring increased clerical salaries associated with maintaining this activity base. The increased cost of gathering data must be weighed against any benefits derived from the added information. Unless benefits are greater to generate than costs, such information should not be gathered.

Identifying service cost centers and their allocation bases is generally based upon Medicare cost report requirements (see Chapter VII, Figure 7.4). Hospitals may identify more cost centers than those required by Medicare and select different allocation bases for internal reporting, using the newly found information to better price goods and services.

Once allocation bases have been selected and activity statistics have been accumulated, the allocation process can begin. This process can be performed manually using step allocation techniques.

A sample step allocation problem follows. While it is not necessary for readers to become adept at the actual process, it is necessary to understand its underlying principles and to be able to interpret its outcome.

This example includes three service and two revenue-producing departments. Listed below are the direct costs that have been charged to each department during the normal course of operations.

Administration	$ 10,000
Maintenance	$ 8,000
Laundry	$ 12,000
Laboratory	$ 55,000
Nursing—Medical Unit	$ 25,000
Total	$110,000

After reviewing relevant information, the following cost allocations bases were determined to be appropriate.

Cost Center	Allocation Base
Administration	Total accumulated costs
Maintenance	Square footage
Laundry	Pounds of clean linen distributed

Statistics gathered for these cost centers appear in Figure 13.1. Accumulated costs, another name for total direct costs, are furnished with the original information.

The order in which cost centers are allocated is important. They should be allocated in the order of most comprehensive coverage. Administration benefits all of the hospital; it should be allocated first. After administration, maintenance serves all of the departments of the institution. Finally, in ordering departments, laundry is listed last because it benefits fewer departments than the others. Figure 13.1 lists the statistics needed for the cost allocation.

After the allocation order has been determined, ratios are established using the selected bases as divisors. These ratios identify the service department cost per unit of service given. The costs of the

	Square Footage	Pounds of Laundry
Administration	1,000	-0-
Maintenance	1,000	100
Laundry	2,000	-0-
Laboratory	3,000	1,000
Nursing Unit	9,000	3,000

Figure 13.1. Statistics needed for cost allocation.

nonrevenue-producing departments are then allocated by applying unit cost to the units of service rendered to each of the following departments. The step method theory states that once a cost center has been allocated, it cannot receive additional allocations from other departments. The object of the process is to allocate all service department costs to the revenue-producing departments. The process is finished when they are the only remaining departments with costs.

After the first service department has been allocated, subsequent service department costs will include direct costs and any costs that were allocated from previously closed service departments.

The results of the allocation are displayed in Figure 13.2. The step allocation process identifies costs associated with providing services and can be interpreted to mean that it costs $75,350 to operate this nursing station and $34,650 to operate the laboratory. Of these costs, $55,000 and $25,000 are direct departmental charges. Each department has been charged these amounts and departmental managers are responsible for controlling these costs. The additional $20,350 ($5,500 + $3,300 + $11,550) for nursing and $9,650 ($2,500 + $3,300 + $3,850) for laboratory are allocated costs or general hospital overhead. General hospital overhead may also be referred to as indirect overhead and is the cost associated with keeping all parts of a hospital running. Revenue-producing department managers cannot be held directly accountable for their allocated cost. Hospital administration accepts responsibility for making service centers efficient contributors and keeping their costs in line with overall revenues.

If a computer is available, the hospital may allocate costs using simultaneous equations. The effect of simultaneous equations is to allocate costs from each service department to all benefitting service departments. An example of simultaneous equations using two departments is provided in Figure 13.3. It is far too complex to use simultaneous equations for more than two departments without computer assistance.

	Service Departments			Revenue-producers	
	Administration	**Maintenance**	**Laundry**	**Nursing**	**Laboratory**
Cost	$10,000	$8,000	$12,000	$55,000	$25,000
Admin.	(10,000)	+ 800	+ 1,200	+5,500	+2,500
Maint.	-0-	(8,800)	+ 2,200	+3,300	+3,300
Laundry			($15,400)	+11,550	+3,850
Total				$75,350	$34,650

Figure 13.2. Results of the allocation.

Now that total costs have been found for the two service departments, their costs can be allocated to the revenue-producing departments.

This allocation process gives management total operating costs by revenue-producing departments, information that can be useful for pricing decisions. If allocated costs are reported at the departmental level, it is important to remember that the reason is not one of accountability but one of pricing. Information concerning allocated costs, if reported, should be separated from direct department costs (see Figure 13.4).

This analysis can be taken further and related to this unit's activity base, making it possible to determine its cost per unit of service. For example, if weighted patient days are the activity base for nursing and there were 900 weighted patient days accumulated by this unit for the month, the cost per weighted patient day would be $83.72 ($75,350 divided by 900). This cost becomes the foundation for determining a reasonable fee for service.

SUMMARY

The institution can be divided into two types of departments: revenue-producing and nonrevenue-producing. Because the fees for service must cover all costs, it is necessary to allocate the costs of nonrevenue-producing departments to the revenue departments that they serve. An activity base or method for allocation must be determined. The more closely the activity base adopted relates to the activity of the nonrevenue-producing department, the more realistic the final answer.

This information is necessary for pricing decisions. It is also beneficial to the process of identifying alternative courses of action, such as choosing between an in-house dietary service and outside catering.

Depts.	Maintenance	Laundry	Surgery	Lab	Total
Costs	$ 8,000	$10,000	$37,000	$44,000	$99,000
Sq. Feet	500	1,500	5,000	3,000	10,000
Laundry	10%		60%	30%	100%

Let L = Laundry
Let M = Maintenance

Total Cost Equations for Each Department
M = $8,000 + 10% of Laundry's Cost

L = $10,000 + 15% (1,500/10,000) of Maintenance's Cost

Therefore:

M = $8,000 + 10% ($10,000 + 15%M)
M = $9,000 + .015M
.985M = $9,000
M = $9,137

And

L = $10,000 + 15% (1,500/10,000) of Maintenance's Cost
L = $10,000 + 15% ($9,137)
L = $11,371

Now that total costs have been found for the two service departments, their costs can be allocated to the revenue-producing departments.

Figure 13.3. Example of simultaneous equation cost allocation.

QUESTIONS

1. What is the difference between allocating costs and charging costs directly to a department?
2. What are the benefits of allocating costs over charging costs to a department?
3. Is the department responsible for its allocated costs?
4. What is overhead?
5. What is the difference between direct and indirect overhead in the context of this text?
6. What is the importance of the allocation base that is selected by a department? What considerations must be given to selecting a base?

Monthly Financial Statement for Nursing

Salaries	$42,000
Supplies	10,000
Other	3,000
Total Direct Costs	$55,000

Allocated Costs

Administration	5,500
Maintenance	3,300
Laundry	11,550
Total Allocated Costs	20,350
Total Departmental Costs	$75,350

Figure 13.4. Information concerning allocated costs should be separated from direct department costs.

7. What is the purpose of cost allocation?
8. What distinguishes a nonrevenue-producing department from one that is revenue-producing? Give an example of each.
9. Why does the order in which departments are allocated have an affect on the outcome? What order should be used?

EXERCISES

1. Hospital Y has two revenue-producing departments (A and B) and two nonrevenue-producing departments (1 and 2). Allocate Department 1 based upon square footage and Department 2 based upon number of employees.

Departments	1	2	A	B	Total
	$1,000	$2,000	$6,000	$8,000	$17,000
Square Footage	100	200	350	450	1,100
Employees	2	3	8	12	25

2. Recalculate #1 if the order of allocation is reversed and Department 2 is allocated first.

XIV

Cost Accounting

CHAPTER OBJECTIVES

1. Define product cost components.
2. Define overhead and explain its relationship to product cost.
3. Introduce standard costing techniques.
4. Explain methodology for isolating variances.
5. Discuss philosophies supporting the creation of standards.
6. Explain how standards can simplify budgeting.

Cost accounting is a discipline that concentrates on identifying and isolating the cost of producing goods and services. Once costs are determined, an institution can determine and evaluate its pricing structure. In those instances where cost exceeds the acceptable price, institutions may choose to eliminate services or find lower-cost alternative goods.

Product/Service Cost Components

It is important to define the cost components of a product or service so that these costs can be identified and attached to the unit produced. Accounting states that product or service cost includes the following:

1. Direct materials incorporated in or used directly in the production of the end good or service,
2. Direct labor involved in making the unit or providing the service, and
3. Overhead, or indirect product costs, the name given to all other production costs, specifically those associated with maintaining

the workplace in which direct materials and direct labor can be combined.

Of these three components, overhead is the most difficult to visualize as a product cost because its impact is not as obvious as direct material and direct labor. Overhead costs include all nondirect materials such as supplies and materials of inconsequential price. It also includes nondirect labor costs such as managerial, transportation, and clerical salaries if these costs are needed to facilitate the production process. Finally, it includes the other costs associated with operating the revenue-producing department, such as equipment and building depreciation, insurance, utilities, and employee benefits for the department, as well as all of the costs of nonrevenue-producing departments not involved in the actual production or patient-service process.

Because it is difficult to visualize, overhead is difficult to trace directly to the product. Whereas direct materials and direct labor can be readily identified with a specific product, overhead costs cannot. Due to the impossibility or impracticality of charging each overhead cost individually, overhead is accumulated for the home department (see Chapter X) and then is allocated or assigned to the product.

The allocation process begins with the determination of a suitable allocation or activity base for charging overhead to the product. The allocation base may vary from one department to the next, and from one company to another, but it should represent a good link between the way that a department's overhead increases and this base unit. For example, many companies use direct labor hours or direct labor dollars as their allocation base because total overhead costs appear to increase as direct labor hours or costs increase. Direct labor hours and dollars are also frequently used because there is no added cost associated with gathering the data since both numbers are readily available in the payroll department.

Practicality aside, the theoretical accuracy of using this base is valid if the industry in question is highly labor-intensive. For those industries that are highly automated, machine hours may be a better indicator for how overhead costs should be allocated to the product. Use of an allocation base other than payroll hours or dollars requires additional work gathering data such as machine hours used during the specific time period and then determining the number of machine hours used to produce each product.

The overhead application rate, or the dollar amount of overhead allocated to the product with each base unit consumed, should be determined at the beginning of the year if it is to be of any benefit to the institution. Because the allocation rate is determined before actual costs have been incurred, it must be based on estimates. Estimates are necessary because product costs must be determined as goods are produced or services provided. Also, overhead costs will vary monthly or sometimes even weekly. For example, utility bills associated with winter months are higher than those of spring and autumn. By using an estimated cost for the year, high and low cost periods can be averaged together. This would keep an institution from establishing one rate for services provided during winter months and another price for services provided in the spring.

The following formula provides the method for determining the estimated overhead rate per base unit of activity.

$$\frac{\text{Estimated Overhead for the Year}}{\text{Estimated Units of Base Measure for the Year}}$$

For example, if the total estimated overhead for 1991 is $100,000 and the estimated direct labor hours are 10,000, and direct labor hours is the base that the institution has selected for applying overhead to the product, then the estimated overhead cost per direct labor hour is $10. Another way of stating the overhead rate is that for every direct labor hour associated with producing a good or service, overhead of $10 will be charged to the product.

METHODS FOR ACCUMULATING COSTS BY PRODUCT OR SERVICE

Manufacturing companies have been coping with the task of identifying product costs for decades. A review of the methods that they are using is beneficial to health care professionals because one of these techniques may be useful in the task of defining health care costs.

Manufacturing companies use two distinct methods or processes for accumulating product costs: 1) job costing and 2) process costing. In some instances, one company will use both methods for the same product, or it may use job costing for some products and process costing for others.

Companies select which method they will use based upon both accuracy and practicality. A good cost accounting system must furnish reliable information without imposing undue burden on information

---

$$\frac{\text{Total costs for the department}}{\text{Total charges for the department}} \times \text{Specific charge for service} = \text{Cost of service}$$

Figure 14.1. The formula for converting charges to costs.

gatherers. For that reason, nurse executives should question whether the value of information gathered is worth the resources used to gather it.

Job Costing

Job costing views each product produced as a unique, individual unit comprised of a unique number of parts or material and which requires its own labor components. Because of its uniqueness, each job is given the status of a cost center, and materials and labor are charged directly to the item produced.

There is a great deal of information accumulated for each job. Therefore, this method is best used where the dollar value of each product warrants the extra work, and each unit can be recognized by its uniqueness. In a hospital setting, each patient could be likened to a job in this costing system. Of course there are some obvious exceptions, the foremost of which is that patients are not viewed as inventory items. The second exception regards items that are being accumulated. The job order cost system accumulates costs by item, whereas patient billing accumulates charges for services by patients. There does not appear to be an efficient system for posting costs to patients' bills. Those institutions that determine a form of job order costing would work for them must recast or convert charges to costs. One way to accomplish this is through the use of ratios. Figure 14.1 gives the formula for converting charges to costs.

For example, for a department whose costs and charges total $100,000 and $120,000, respectively, the cost of a service charged out at $90 would be $75 ($100,000/$120,000 × $90). Using ratio analysis to identify costs is based upon the assumption that the department uses a standard percentage markup on costs. Since the cost of the item is what the institution is trying to identify, this assumption may prove to be an inherent flaw for most departments. Using a job order system to determine product costs will only be valid to the extent that departments use uniform markup rates.

Given this limitation, there are still valid applications for job cost-ing techniques within an institution. This system would work for those central service and orthopedic units that can identify direct material costs. A standard markup can then be used to cover the department's overhead and allow for some profit.

For those departments that do not lend themselves well to job order costing, process costing may be a viable alternative for determin-ing product cost.

Process Costing

Process costing is used by manufacturers of relatively low-cost and/or multiple, homogenous goods. In these settings, practicality prohibits maintaining cost records for each item produced. Therefore production costs (direct materials, direct labor, and overhead) are charged to the producing department rather than to the job. Periodically, production costs are accumulated and spread over all units produced, thus identi-fying the cost per unit.

In those departments where more than one good or service is pro-duced, management must develop a common denominator for units produced. This common denominator is often referred to as a relative value unit (RVU). The process of assigning RVUs to services necessi-tates identifying the simplest unit of work and then redefining all other services in relation to this base unit. For example, if direct labor is a good indicator of relative value and unit A requires one labor hour while unit B requires two hours to complete, and if this department produces 100 As and 100 Bs, the RVUs of work produced is 300 (as shown in Figure 14.2).

How this example is applied to individual institutions will depend on their organization. Some institutions have organized their opera-tions according to product lines. Such an institution could have a prod-uct line entitled "Women's Health" in which obstetric deliveries are accounted for as complete cost units. Such an organization would ac-cumulate costs from many supporting departments under the heading of normal delivery, and may have a standard fee for the service pro-vided that encompasses all of the supporting costs.

Other institutions may have traditional organizations where nurs-ing units provide continuous care, but the patient travels to other de-partments to obtain laboratory, radiology, delivery, and surgical services. The service revenue and costs for these other departments

	Number of units	×	Relative value/unit	=	Total relative value
A	100	×	1	=	100
B	100	×	2	=	<u>200</u>
					<u>300</u>

Figure 14.2. Calculating relative value per unit.

remain in the servicing unit and the nursing unit receives revenue for the room charges only. The institution's organizational structure will determine which costs become part of the product and how it is billed.

The analogy for the example might be applied to either system with "A" representing normal deliveries (in total for the product line institution and day rate charges for the maternity nursing unit model) and "B" representing deliveries with accompanying complications. The example has been simplified in units and amounts to illustrate the concepts.

Patient DRGs may form the basis for developing RVUs for institutions organized by product lines, and patient acuity levels may form the basis for nursing unit RVUs. For comparison between nursing units, a standardized system should be used that can be applied to maternity and intensive care alike. Similar RVUs should be developed for ancillary units such as laboratory, respiratory therapy, etc. The development of unit costs occurs in reverse. First, costs are accumulated for the following categories: material and supplies, direct labor, and overhead, both variable and fixed. Then the RVU base is applied to the patients served during the period. The total accumulated costs is then divided by the RVU to determine the cost per base RVU.

To extend the previous example, if costs, including estimated overhead, for the unit total $4,500, then the cost per RVU is $1.50 ($4,500 divided by 300). The cost assigned to product A is $1.50 (number of RVUs/unit × cost per RVU), while $3.00 become the cost of B. The greater the variety of goods and services produced by the department, the more time-consuming the original weighing process becomes. The key factor lies in initially determining a reasonably accurate RVU. Once established, the scheme of weights must be reviewed and updated as procedures, and therefore RVUs, change. The initial process of determining RVUs may have been standardized by the profession as it has been for laboratory procedures or it may require expertise from outside the department. Systems or industrial engineers may be called in to help departments devise a schedule of RVUs. If outside expertise is used, it is essential that managers furnish the necessary guidance that will give outsiders an understanding of the internal operations of the unit.

Computers facilitate the mechanical process of tabulating and accumulating RVUs once a system is in place. The tabulation becomes a simple by-product of departmental revenue summaries.

Cost accounting techniques require the accumulation of costs individually by patient or collectively by either DRG or processes (departments) to determine whether the institution is operating profitably. Institutions may use both job costing and process costing to accumulate their product costs.

One accounting tool that many hospitals have adopted to help them with the task of cost accounting and evaluating operations is standard costing. Standard costing requires further analysis of each specific service to determine its components.

Standard Costing

Both job order and process costing take a historical perspective and report what actual product costs were incurred for the period. There is a technique used by manufacturing concerns that analyzes the product and specifies what its input requirements should be. It further costs out the inputs. This additional information can be used to evaluate monthly performance as well as to budget future expenditures. For example, Figure 14.3 shows the standard material and labor costs associated with producing "A."

Actual production information for the period reveals that 1,000 units of A were produced and that the following resources were used during production:

Material	2,200 units of input	$3,400
Labor	600 hours	5,400

Managers can analyze why actual costs are $8,800 rather than the projected $8,000 (1,000 units @ $8.00 per unit). Figure 14.4 shows how variance analysis can be used to isolate the usage variances that arise from using units of input other than the amount called for by the standard. Usage variances can be separated from price variances (the name given to the difference generated by paying a different amount

Item	Input	Cost/unit of input	Total Cost
Material	2 units	$1.50/unit	$3.00
Labor	½ hour	$10.00/hour	5.00
		Total	$8.00

Figure 14.3. Standards for producing Product A.

for the input resource than that which was specified by the standard). The reason and nature of the variance must be identified. A "U" is assigned to those variances where the cost is greater than that specified by the standard. "U" denotes that the variance is unfavorable. An "F"

MATERIAL

Actual units of input @ actual price/unit	3,400	
Actual units of input @ standard price/unit		
(2,200 @ $1.50)	3,300	
Material Price Variance		$100 U
Actual units of input @ standard price/unit		
(2,200 @ $1.50)	3,300	
Standard units of input @ standard price/unit		
(1,000 completed units @ 2 units each		
or 2,000 @ $1.50)	3,000	
Material Usage Variance		$300 U

LABOR

Actual units of input @ actual price/unit	5,400	
Actual units of input @ standard price/unit		
(600 hours @ $10.00)	6,000	
Labor Rate Variance		$600 F
Actual units of input @ standard price/unit		
(600 hours @ $10.00)	6,000	
Standard units of input @ standard price/unit		
(1,000 completed units @ ½ hours each		
or 500 hrs. @ $10.00)	5,000	
Labor Efficiency Variance		$1,000 U

Figure 14.4. Variance analysis for material and labor.

is assigned to favorable variances where costs are less than what the standard specifies.

Labor Given this information, managers can identify the reasons why costs were different than planned. For example, using the information from Figure 14.4, the managers can explain the $800 difference between actual costs and standard costs in terms of the following variances:

Material Price Variance	$ 100 U
Material Usage Variance	300 U
Labor Rate Variance	600 F
Labor Efficiency Variance	1,000 U
Difference between Actual and Standard Costs	$ 800 U

Armed with this information, managers can identify the source of the problems. Material cost problems are beyond the realm of most managers to solve because these variances belong to the purchasing department. To a certain extent, labor rate variances are also beyond the control of managers unless they can effectively shift work loads to accomplish the substitution of less expensive labor for higher paid services. In many instances this may not be possible.

Material usage and labor efficiency variances can be investigated and the cause of the variance identified. If a problem exists it can be corrected by controlling inventory usage or initiating procedural changes. As in other matters, managers must be able to identify the problem before attempts can be made to solve it.

Overhead Analysis

Once direct material and direct labor variances have been analyzed, managers should analyze overhead variances. As mentioned previously, overhead is the name given to all other costs associated with operating the institution. Managers can only analyze the overhead variances for their departments. Before beginning this operation, overhead must be separated by cost behavior pattern. Fixed overhead must be separated from variable overhead (see Chapter VIII) .

Standards should incorporate costs for these two product cost elements. Since overhead is generally applied to a product based upon

VARIABLE OVERHEAD

Actual units of input @ actual price/unit	$5,000	
Actual units of input @ standard price/unit		
(600 hours @ $9.00)	<u>5,400</u>	
Variable Overhead Spending Variance		$400 F
Actual units of input @ standard price/unit		
(600 hours @ $9.00)	5,400	
Standard units of input @ standard price/unit		
(1,000 completed units		
@ 1/2 hours each or 500 hrs. @ $9.00)	<u>4,500</u>	
Variable Overhead Efficiency Variance		$900 U

Figure 14.5. Variance analysis for variable overhead.

using direct labor as its base, the standard may refer to hours of variable overhead charged to the product. Variable overhead may also be related directly to direct labor cost and stated as a percent of direct labor cost.

Expanding the previous example to include overhead cost components might yield the following standard:

Variable Overhead   1/2 hour @ $9.00/hour $4.50

The variable overhead rate is calculated using the formula for determining the estimated overhead rate per base unit of activity, which was discussed previously. Standard variable overhead, or the variable overhead that should have been incurred at the present level of activity, can then be compared to the actual costs of $5,000 for variable overhead that were incurred for the period. Figure 14.5 prepares an analysis of standard and actual variable overhead costs similar to that prepared for material and direct labor.

Variable overhead is the total of many individual cost items. Because variable overhead is applied based upon direct labor hours, controlling direct labor hours will control the variable overhead efficiency variance. The variable overhead spending variance results from spending more for those variable overhead items than was originally planned. This spending variance may be partly the responsibility of the department but it may also rest in part with other departments. Institutions need to decide how detailed the analysis of standard variances will be and department lines may need to be crossed in the name of controlling costs. For example, office supplies, utilities, patient transportation, and laundry are a few of the variable costs of a unit. Depending on the internal cost accounting and reporting system, managers may have different levels of knowledge regarding all of the unit's variable costs. At minimum, the managers should be aware of the variable overhead costs that are directly used and charged to the unit. This information can be analyzed in a fashion similar to that identified in Figure 14.5. Once that has been accomplished, managers can gather information concerning all other variable costs that are allocated to the unit. This information may already be available and included in the monthly financial statements that are distributed to the unit. If this information is not currently provided, the information can be obtained from the finance department. A management team should review these allocations to determine if they are reasonable and to spot unusual changes that occur over time or between hospital departments. The more informed managers become, the better they are able to help their institution identify problems and to recommend alternatives.

Fixed overhead costs also exist, but these costs cannot be controlled in the short run. Fixed overhead costs include the salaries of administration, depreciation costs of the building and equipment being used, property and malpractice insurance, and other similar types of costs. The level of fixed costs for any given institution will depend upon anticipated activity levels and the required resources necessary to support that level. Once committed to a level of activity, the fixed costs associated with operations should not vary from one period to the next. These types of costs are generally beyond the scope of most managers to change or affect from one period to the next.

USING STANDARDS FOR BUDGETING _____

Institutions that have adopted standard costing will find it easier to budget for future operations. The standard is a prediction of what the product or service cost should be broken by cost component. To budget for operations, managers need to take the total budgeted services and multiply each service by the material cost component to determine supply cost and by labor cost components to determine labor costs. Such analysis can serve as a baseline for budgeting operations. For example, if the standard material costs for product A are 2 units @ $1.50, and the costs are expected to increase 10% with the expected number of procedures estimated at 100 per month, then the materials budgeted for each month for this product are $3,300 or 100 @ $3.30.

Philosophy Behind Standards

At this point it is important to identify the institution's philosophy supporting its standards. There are currently three different philosophies being used by industry. They include the following.

1. Ideal Standards—norms for inputs and costs based upon the best possible performance under existing operating conditions.
2. Currently Attainable Standards—norms for inputs and costs based upon best possible performance with allowances for some idleness, breakdowns, and losses.
3. Average Past Performance Standards—norms of input and costs based upon the results of previous operations.

If a system of standard costing is being used, it is essential that managers understand its underlying premise. If the institution adopted the philosophy of making ideal standards, it must realize that this will always yield unfavorable variances, because the workplace is not populated with robots who always perform the same task in the same way. Individuals cannot sustain indefinite periods of peak performance, nor is the hospital a setting that dictates that each patient will respond in exactly the same manner to the same procedure. Standard costing should be used to encourage and motivate employees to do their best as human beings. Reports that constantly display unfavorable variances may have the opposite effect on the employees. Conversely, developing standards based upon the status quo may build slack and waste into the system, and fail to achieve cost control goals. For that reason, it makes sense to develop standards based upon currently attainable goals. Such standards incorporate some breaks in the work load and allow for differences that may exist from one patient to another. Such standards serve to motivate employees to do their best while identifying problems as they occur.

SUMMARY

Managers can learn many lessons in product cost accounting from for-profit companies. Understanding the various cost accounting methodologies and techniques that are available can help nurse executives design, implement, and use a cost accounting system that will identify the costs associated with products and services provided. Standard costing systems also serve as valuable tools for budgeting, evaluating, and controlling departmental costs. In those instances where they are useful, they furnish important information that is necessary for pricing products, determining alternatives or substitute services, and controlling costs.

QUESTIONS

1. What costs are defined as product costs? How do product costs differ from allocated costs?
2. Define the term overhead. Does overhead differ depending on the department in question?
3. Why is overhead allocated rather than charged directly to a product or service?
4. What is a product standard? How can standards help managers plan, control, and evaluate operations? Who determines a product's standard?
5. Explain the different philosophies that can dictate the components of a standard.
6. What is job costing? Give examples of when job costing is applicable for product costing. Give examples of when job costing can be used in the hospital environment.
7. What is process costing? How does it differ from job costing?

EXERCISES

1. Hospital A has developed a standard for Procedure X. It is listed below.

Labor	1 hour @ $15/hour
Supplies	2 units @ $2 each

Actual procedures performed during the month total 1,000 and the following costs were incurred for the item.

Labor	1,100 hours	$15,750
Supplies	2,100 units	$ 4,500

Isolate the labor rate and efficiency variances and the material price and usage variances. Explain what procedures would be used to follow up on each variance.

2. What budget would be prepared if this department planned to perform 1,677 procedures in a given month?
3. What is the overhead application rate if overhead is applied on the basis of direct labor hours, given the following information.

Estimated
- Overhead $100,000
- Direct Labor hours 25,000
- Direct Labor cost $450,000

Actual
- Overhead $111,000
- Direct Labor hours 27,235
- Direct Labor Cost $589,133

XV

Decision Making

CHAPTER OBJECTIVES

1. Define and identify relevant information necessary for decision making.
2. Distinguish revenue-generating decisions from cost-saving decisions.
3. Describe a methodology that can be used for management decisions.

Operating decisions are made daily. Some such operating decisions are outlined below.

1. Deciding whether to contract with outside vendors or provide the service internally.
2. Pricing new products or services.
3. Deciding whether fees will be discounted in exchange for increased volume.

While each of these decisions is different in detail and scope, they can all be resolved using similar techniques.

Gathering Relevant Information

The first step in the decision-making process is to identify all available alternatives. This step involves a certain amount of brainstorming and no alternative should be dismissed at this early stage.

Managers must then gather relevant information supporting each alternative. Relevant information is defined as any financial data that will change or differ depending on the course of action or alternative selected. Use the following example to identify all relevant information.

Example

    Hospital X currently owns and operates a laundry. A private contractor has agreed to pick up, launder, and return clean linen to the hospital for a fixed fee of $20,000 a month plus $0.10 per pound of clean laundry returned. The contractor promises a two-day turn-around time. Hospital X currently launders 150,000 pounds of linen a month. Annual operating costs for the last fiscal year follow.

Salaries, supervisory	$ 60,000
Salaries, laundry workers	300,000
Salaries, distribution	120,000
Linen	100,000
Cleaning supplies	50,000
Repairs and maintenance	20,000
Other	10,000
Total	$660,000

    Figure 15.1 identifies the relevant information for the two alternatives of contracting with the outside vendor or providing the service internally.

    If the outside vendor's contract is accepted, the hospital will be able to eliminate all departmental costs except $25,000 of supervisory salaries, $100,000 of linen costs, and $120,000 of distribution salaries.

    To identify relevant information, one must first identify all alternatives. In this example, there are two alternatives: 1) keep the hospital laundry, or 2) close it and contract with an outside vendor. The relevant information for this problem will be that information that changes between alternatives.

    An analysis of relevant information shows that Hospital X would save $5,000 annually by operating its own laundry. There may be other relevant information outside of the department's cost report that should be considered. Such pertinent information includes useful life and expected maintenance of present equipment, other potential uses for the laundry space, length of time covered by the vendor contract, and constancy of the pricing schedule. Some qualitative factors may also influence decisions. They may include the following:

	Keep Department	Outside Vendor
Salaries, supervisory	$ 35,000	-0-
Salaries	300,000	-0-
Cleaning supplies	50,000	-0-
Repairs and maintenance	20,000	-0-
Other	10,000	-0-
Contract cost/year		
Fixed fee ($20,000 × 12)		$240,000
Variable cost		
(150,000 pounds × $0.10/ pound		
× 12 months	-0-	180,000
Total costs	$415,00	$420,000

Figure 15.1. Relevant information for deciding whether to contract with an outside vendor or to provide the service internally.

1. The vendor's reputation for reliability and work performance,
2. Employment opportunities available for current laundry employees that could be displaced by the change,
3. The effect that closing a hospital department could have on employee morale, and
4. The existence of other viable alternatives besides the two considered, especially if the new vendor is selected and might later prove unable to meet the hospital's requirements.

Business decisions should not be based entirely upon the bottom line. Qualitative factors may influence the final decision away from the alternative with the greatest savings. In that case, managers must be aware of all added costs that are being accepted because of qualitative factors.

Other Business Decisions

Business decisions may involve adding and pricing a new service. Fees charged should cover all costs of providing the new service. First, those costs must be identified.

Costs are charged directly to revenue-producing departments. These costs fall into two categories, direct product costs and overhead. Cost of resources used in the actual performance of the service is called product cost. Laboratory technician salaries and laboratory supplies are examples of product costs.

Other departmental expenses, not directly used when performing a service are called overhead. These expenses are necessary for the efficient operation of the department and include such items as clerical salaries and office supplies. Overhead may also include supervisory salaries if a supervisor's responsibilities include ordering supplies, scheduling and supervising employees, and evaluating their performance. At those times when supervisors work directly on patient tests, their salaries become part of the product cost.

In addition to direct departmental costs, there are other costs that must be covered by fees for service. Nonrevenue-producing departments are necessary to its efficient operation, and are therefore part of overhead. These costs are allocated to revenue-producing departments to identify total department costs. They are not charged directly to the unit (see Chapter XIII).

Demand

When a new service is being contemplated, hospitals begin by forecasting future demand for the service. Physicians are polled to determine its potential use. Medical records can also serve as an information source. Demand can be forecasted by reviewing medical cases where this procedure would have been used had it existed at the time.

For explanatory purposes, suppose that a laboratory is considering offering a new procedure. Financial data concerning this test is furnished in Figure 15.2.

To establish a fee for this service, a manager must also gather departmental operating information. The laboratory's monthly income statement is given in Figure 15.3. It has been reformatted to separate direct departmental costs into product and departmental or indirect overhead. Hospital overhead allocated to the department is referred to as indirect overhead.

Since this department is using cost as its basis for pricing, relationships must be established based upon direct product costs ($80,000) and direct departmental overhead ($10,000). Direct departmental overhead is 12 ½% of direct product costs.

Technician time (15 minutes @ $10.00/hour)	$2.50
Supplies	1.50
Total product cost of procedure	$4.00

Figure 15.2. Financial data for a new laboratory test.

If a hospital wants to be consistent when establishing fees, based upon existent cost relationships, it will add 12 ½% to base product costs to cover departmental overhead. It will also add 25% (allocated costs of $20,000 divided by product costs of $80,000 = 25%) to the base cost to cover indirect overhead. The new procedure's adjusted cost becomes $5.50 (Figure 15.4). A hospital will also include a profit element in its fee. This profit is necessary to ensure that there will be additional funds available to support continued operations. If this entity decided that it needed to generate $1,000 profit from this service, and demand is forecasted at 1,000 tests per month, it would add $1.00 to the $5.50 total costs and arrive at a final fee of $6.50.

Only tests performed on those patients who pay full charges generate profit. Government program outpatients pay the lower of cost or charges. Specific insurance carriers may have been given discounts through preferred provider contracts. Both of these instances will reduce the overall profitability of the new test.

Laboratory Revenues	$112,000
Direct Departmental Costs	
Product Costs	
Salaries	55,000
Supplies	20,000
Other	5,000
Overhead	
Supervisory, clerical	
salaries and other	
miscellaneous expenses	10,000
Direct departmental income	22,000
Allocated or indirect overhead	20,000
Net income for department	$ 2,000

Figure 15.3. Laboratory income statement.

Direct product cost of performing test	$4.00
Direct departmental overhead	
(12 1/2% of $4.00)	.50
Indirect departmental overhead	
(25% of $4.00)	1.00
Total costs	$5.50

Figure 15.4. Calculation of the new procedure's adjusted cost.

If a hospital must realize an average profit of $1.00 per test, it will need to estimate the number of tests that will be performed for discounted groups. To continue this example, this hospital estimates that 1,000 tests will be performed monthly. Of this number, 40% or 400 are expected to be completed for Medicare and Medicaid patients. These 400 patients yield no profit. It is therefore up to the 600 full-charge paying patients to generate the $1,000 profit. To realize a total profit of $1,000, the hospital must set its fee at $7.17 (see Figure 15.5).

Special Pricing Arrangements

A hospital may enter into a contract with an HMO (Health Maintenance Organization) or an insurance carrier to furnish tests and procedures to their members at reduced fees. The terms of the agreement may stipulate that a specific number of tests would be purchased annually. Managers would be wise to accept a discounted fee for service arrangements if it will increase total profits.

Total profit need (1,000 tests @ $1.00/test)	$1,000
Profit generated by government program patients	-0-
Profit to be derived by self-pay patients	$1,000
Number of procedures that must generate the	
profit (60% of 1,000)	600
Profit added to costs ($1,000 / 600)	$1.67
Total costs of procedure	5.50
Proposed fee	$7.17

Figure 15.5. Calculation of the new procedure's cost, including discounts for government program patients.

	Accept	Reject
Revenues		
(200 @ $5.00)	$1,000	-0-
Added Costs		
Salaries (200 @ $2.50)	(500)	-0-
Supplies (200 @ $1.50)	(300)	-0-
Additional income	$ 200	-0-

Figure 15.6. Analysis of incremental cost and revenue.

A hospital will increase total profits as long as discounted fees are greater than the additional or incremental product costs associated with providing each test. Incremental product costs are any product costs that will increase as a direct result of doing the extra tests. By definition, incremental costs will be total variable costs associated with the test. Fixed costs may also be included but only if these fixed costs must be added to attain the new volume of service.

Incremental costs are those costs that are added as a direct result of the contract being accepted. To return to the laboratory pricing problem, the incremental cost associated with one laboratory procedure is $4.00, the labor and supply cost of doing one test. Even though overhead, both direct and indirect, are costs of doing business and are included in the fee, normal operations have already covered these costs. Acceptance of this contract should not add to these costs. If overhead does increase as a direct result of added work load, then that incremental overhead cost (the amount of the increase) should be included to determine the minimum fee that the hospital would be willing to accept and not negatively affect existing profits.

If an HMO agrees to pay $5.00 for each test, and guarantees a monthly volume of 200 tests, management should agree to the contract because the arrangement will yield it an additional profit of $200 (see Figure 15.6).

There are qualitative considerations in accepting a special pricing agreement. Other insurance carriers may learn of it and demand similar discounts. The HMO may not be generating new business for the hospital, but in fact be receiving a discount on services for which it had been paying full charges under a different reimbursement arrangement. Once a discounted arrangement has been agreed to, there is little likelihood that the HMO will ever pay full charges again.

Equipment Acquisitions

Equipment purchases are an intricate part of cost saving and revenue generating decisions. A hospital should purchase equipment if it will generate operating revenue or save future period costs. Relevant information for equipment acquisition decisions include the following.

1. Anticipated number of procedures to be performed annually
2. Anticipated fee for service
3. Incremental cost of providing service
4. Equipment cost, including delivery and installation charges
5. Expected useful life of equipment
6. Expected salvage or residual value of equipment on the last day of its useful life
7. Expected repairs and maintenance costs over the asset's life

The information needed relates to costs and revenues that will change with each alternative (accept or reject). Equipment acquisition decisions are especially difficult because the asset is long-lived. A hospital is therefore committing funds for much longer periods of time when it decides to purchase fixed assets. The next chapter will address unique techniques that can be used to further analyze fixed asset acquisitions. The relevant data-gathering techniques discussed in this chapter will be the starting point for further analysis.

When considering replacing an existing machine, acquisition costs associated with existing machinery are irrelevant to the replacement decision because these costs will not change between the alternatives of buying or not buying. However, information concerning existing equipment may be useful insofar as it furnishes estimates that can be used to predict future costs or asset life. The decision to replace will be made only if benefits derived from purchasing the new machine are greater than those benefits derived from operating existing equipment.

Example

A hospital owns an X-ray machine that is currently being used to take 3,000 X rays a year. The average charge per X ray is $20. The X-ray machine cost $20,000 new. It has a remaining life of five years and a residual value of $1,000.

A new machine will cost $35,000. It will have a useful life of five years and no residual value at the end of its life. The manufacturer

	Buy New	Keep Old
Changes in expense:		
Expense reduction $5.00		
Annual volume _3,000_		
Annual savings $15,000		
Asset life 5 years		
Total expense reduction	$75,000	-0-
Cost of new equipment $35,000		
Less residual value		
of old machine _1,000_		
Net cost of new machine		
Total savings for 5 years	34,000	
	$41,000	-0-
Average annual savings	$ 8,200	-0-

Figure 15.7. Analysis of a possible purchase of an X-ray machine.

states that the new machine will save $5.00 per procedure because it will use less film and take less time to process. The hospital does not anticipate a change in the level of usage during the next five years.

Analysis of the two alternatives appears in Figure 15.7. Only relevant information has been considered. Zeros are listed under the "keep" alternative to show a base point for savings. The revenue of $60,000 that is to be generated by the test is ignored because it will not change between the two alternatives and is therefore irrelevant to the decision.

Given this information, the hospital should purchase the replacement equipment because that decision will generate a savings of $41,000 over the five-year period.

SUMMARY

Decisions are made by managers every day. The methodology for decision making involves three steps.

1. Identify all viable alternatives.
2. Isolate all relevant information associated with each alternative.
3. Compare net revenue or savings that are generated by each alternative.

Quantitatively, the manager should select the alternative that provides the highest revenue or savings. There are qualitative considerations that are part of every decision. Quantitative factors should be calculated first. Then, if qualitative factors cause a reversal of the original decision, the costs associated with supporting qualitative factors can be determined.

QUESTIONS

1. What is meant by relevant data? Give an example to support your answer.
2. Explain why the cost of the existing equipment is irrelevant to the decision to replace that equipment.
3. Discuss the following statement. "Irrelevant data can either be included in the analysis or ignored. If it is included, it must be included twice."
4. What is meant by incremental cost or revenue? Give an example to support your answer.
5. Distinguish between quantitative and qualitative factors that affect decision making.
6. What are qualitative factors that affect decision making?
7. Give examples of some of the qualitative factors that could affect the decision to computerize a nursing station.
8. Discuss how, when, and to what extent qualitative factors should affect the final decision.

EXERCISES

1. The hospital performs a specific laboratory procedure for which it charges the patient $10. Each year, 7,000 procedures are performed. The annual costs associated with performing this procedure are given below.

	Total annual costs	Per unit costs
Salaries	$14,000	$2.00
Supplies	7,000	1.00
Depreciation	21,000	3.00
General overhead	24,500	3.50
Total	66,500	$9.50

A local HMO has contacted the hospital and has agreed to purchase 1,000 procedures a year for its program participants. The maximum price that the HMO will agree to pay is $8. Should the institution accept the proposal? Explain your answer.

2. The organization has received a request to purchase a new machine that costs $200,000. An old machine that cost $120,000 can be traded in for the new equipment. If that is done, the manufacturer will reduce the invoice price by $2,000. The equipment has a useful life of 10 years. The department has generated the following cost and revenue information for the machine.

New machine will perform 10,000 tests annually.

Fee charged per test	$6
Annual costs to operate:	
Salary of operator	$10,000
Supplies	5,500
Depreciation	20,000

Required: Analyze the information given and decide whether the new machine should be purchased.

3. An alternative exists to purchasing the machine in #2. That is to have the test sample taken in-house and sent to a neighboring laboratory. The costs involved in this alternative are given below.

Annual salary of sample gatherer	$6,000
Supplies	3,500
Fee charged by the laboratory	$4.00

XVI

Capital Budgeting

CHAPTER OBJECTIVES

1. Identify the purpose of capital budgeting.
2. Explain how the relevant information gathered in the last chapter can be modified to reflect the time value of money.
3. Facilitate understanding time value of money concepts, and the mathematical tables that are used in present value calculations.
4. Identify capital budgeting techniques.
5. Identify advantages and disadvantages that are associated with the various capital budgeting techniques.

Decisions involving fixed asset acquisitions are difficult because they generally involve investments of large sums of money for long periods of time. Once made, errors are often very difficult to repair. Because of its specialized nature, it may be impossible to sell the fixed asset or, if sold, only a fraction of the purchase price may be realized. Add to this the fact that hospital resources are limited and there are always more fixed asset requisitions than there are funds with which to purchase them and the importance of making the correct decision becomes imperative. Tools must be developed to help managers choose which fixed assets to buy. Two such tools are payback and net present value.

PAYBACK

Payback is an accounting tool that lets a business calculate how long it will take to recover money spent for equipment.

Payback Formula:

$$\frac{\text{Investment in Equipment}}{\text{Annual net cash generated}} = \frac{\text{Number of years to recoup}}{\text{the initial investment}}$$
(net of costs paid)

Example

Listed below is the information that relates to the purchase of a new machine.

Cost of new equipment	$500,000
Expected useful life	8 years
Estimated value at the end of its life	-0-
Anticipated annual utilization in units	5,000
Fee per procedure (assume no discounts)	$40
Anticipated annual operating costs :	
Salary of operator	$20,000
Supply costs	$10/unit
Utilities	$ 1/unit
Annual Depreciation	$63,333*

*Depreciation is equal to $500,000, divided by 8 years.

Calculation of cash generated each year:

Revenues (5,000 @ $40)		$200,000
Costs		
Salaries	$24,000	
Supplies	50,000	
Utilities	5,000	
Total Costs		79,000
Annual increase in cash		$121,000
Estimated Number of years of use		8
Estimated Total Cash generated		$968,000

(Note that depreciation is not included as a cost because it does not represent a cash payment. Depreciation is the allocation of the cost of a fixed asset to the time periods that it serves.)

Using decision-making techniques from previous chapters, this equipment should be purchased. Total benefits of eight years of oper-

$$\frac{\text{Investment in Equipment}}{\text{Cash generated annually}} = \frac{\$500,000}{121,000} = 4.13 \text{ years}$$

Figure 16.1. Payback calculation.

ation are $968,000, an increase of $468,000 over the out-of-pocket costs.

According to the payback calculation in Figure 16.1, it will take the institution a little over four years to recoup its cash purchase price. This payback formula serves as a screening tool. As long as the payback period is less than the estimated useful life of an asset, equipment purchases will result in a positive net cash inflow.

The longer the payback period, the more likely that outside factors may change, affecting the ultimate outcome of an investment decision. Just the fact that an institution estimates data for many years into the future incorporates an element of uncertainty into its calculations. For that reason, institutions usually require that an arbitrary payback period of five or less years be met.

NET PRESENT VALUE

Simplicity and ease of understanding make payback calculations a valuable screening tool. Its value is diminished, however, because it overlooks an important economic factor; namely, that there is a time value to money. Money in hand today is worth more than money that is expected to be received one year from now. Ignoring the possibility of failure to collect, money in hand today can be reinvested in securities or savings certificates and actually be worth more next year than it is today. Conversely, money to be received at a future date is worth less today because interest earned during the interim holding period does not belong to the potential holder.

Equipment purchase decisions involve cash payments today that are expected to generate greater cash inflows over the life of the asset. Opportunity costs associated with purchasing equipment instead of investing those funds in other more current investment alternatives should be considered. Net present value calculations consider the time value of money and discounts future cash inflows to the value that they would be worth today, thus removing all interest that could have been earned had the cash been on hand today.

	Simple Interest	=	Principal	×	Rate	×	Time
Year 1	$20	=	$200	×	10%	×	1 year
Year 2	20	=	$200	×	10%	×	1 year
Total	$40						

	Compound Interest	=	Principal	×	Rate	×	Time
Year 1	$20	=	$200	×	10%	×	1 year
Year 2	22	=	220	×	10%	×	1 year
Total	$42						

Figure 16.2. Comparison of simple and compound interest.

For example, if an available investment alternative is a savings account that pays 10% annual interest, an institution must invest $0.91 today in order to have $1.00 in the account at the end of the year. The further into the future the money is needed, the lesser the amount that must be invested today and the more interest that is generated.

At a minimum, lending institutions compound interest annually. Generally it is compounded more often. Compounding interest means that banks regularly calculate and pay interest on the principal and interest amounts that have been credited to an account before the day of calculation. Compounding interest permits savings to grow at a faster rate. The more often interest is calculated and added to the base, the faster the rate of growth. Compare the computation of simple interest for two years at 10% per year on $200 to the same computation using compound interest. See Figure 16.2 for a simple comparison of simple and compound interest.

Manually calculating compound interest is a lengthy and cumbersome process. To save time and effort, mathematicians have created a set of mathematical tables, called present value tables, that furnish the same results (Figures 16.3, 16.4). They will enable a reader to calculate the present value of future cash inflows, deducting any interest that would have been included in the future amount. Both present value tables give the present value of one dollar to be received at some future time. To solve a specific problem, a reader need only multiply the factor that is found in the table by the actual number of dollars to be

Periods	6%	8%	10%	12%	14%	16%
1	0.943	0.926	0.909	0.893	0.877	0.833
2	0.890	0.857	0.826	0.797	0.769	0.743
3	0.840	0.794	0.751	0.712	0.675	0.641
4	0.792	0.735	0.683	0.636	0.592	0.552
5	0.747	0.681	0.621	0.567	0.519	0.476
6	0.705	0.630	0.564	0.507	0.456	0.410
7	0.665	0.583	0.513	0.452	0.400	0.354
8	0.627	0.540	0.467	0.404	0.351	0.305
9	0.592	0.500	0.424	0.361	0.308	0.263
10	0.558	0.463	0.386	0.322	0.270	0.227
11	0.527	0.429	0.350	0.287	0.237	0.195
12	0.497	0.397	0.319	0.257	0.208	0.168
13	0.469	0.368	0.290	0.229	0.182	0.145
14	0.442	0.340	0.263	0.205	0.160	0.125
15	0.417	0.315	0.239	0.183	0.140	0.108
16	0.394	0.292	0.218	0.163	0.123	0.093
17	0.371	0.270	0.198	0.146	0.108	0.080
18	0.350	0.250	0.180	0.130	0.095	0.069
19	0.331	0.232	0.164	0.116	0.083	0.060
20	0.312	0.215	0.149	0.104	0.073	0.051

Figure 16.3. Present value of $1: $P = F_n/(1 + r)^n$.

received. For example, using the Present Value of $1 table, the factor associated with 3 periods at 5% interest is 0.864. If $500 is to be received at the end of three years, its present value is $432 if discounted at 5%.

Mathematicians have developed a table to speed the calculation of the present value of multiple receipts. If the same amount is received at regular intervals, this table can be used because it incorporates multiple receipts or payments into the calculation. Annuity is the name given to the receipt of the same amount of money at the end of regular time intervals. Instead of calculating the present value of each receipt and then adding their products, one can multiply the factor for the interest rate and time period that is found in the Present Value of an

Periods	6%	8%	10%	12%	14%	16%
1	0.943	0.926	0.909	0.893	0.877	0.833
2	1.833	1.783	1.736	1.690	1.647	1.605
3	2.673	2.577	2.487	2.402	2.322	2.246
4	3.465	3.312	3.170	3.037	2.914	2.798
5	4.212	3.993	3.791	3.605	3.433	3.274
6	4.917	4.623	4.355	4.111	3.889	3.685
7	5.582	5.206	4.868	4.564	4.288	4.039
8	6.210	5.747	5.335	4.968	4.639	4.344
9	6.802	6.247	5.759	5.328	4.946	4.607
10	7.360	6.710	6.145	5.650	5.216	4.833
11	7.887	7.139	6.495	5.988	5.453	5.029
12	8.384	7.536	6.814	6.194	5.660	5.197
13	8.853	7.904	7.103	6.424	5.842	5.342
14	9.295	8.244	7.367	6.628	6.002	5.468
15	9.712	8.559	7.606	6.811	6.142	5.575
16	10.106	8.851	7.824	6.974	6.265	5.669
17	10.477	9.122	8.022	7.120	6.373	5.749
18	10.828	9.372	8.201	7.250	6.467	5.818
19	11.158	9.604	8.365	7.366	6.550	5.877
20	11.470	9.818	8.514	7.469	6.623	5.929

Figure 16.4. Present value of an ordinary annuity: $P_n = 1/r[1 - 1/(1 + r)^2]$.

Ordinary Annuity of $1 table by the dollar amount that will be received in each period.

For example, if $100 is to be received at the end of each of the next 4 years in a 10% interest market, the present value of the amounts to be received is $316.99. Detailed calculations are furnished in Figure 16.5.

The same answer can be derived by taking the 4 period/10% factor from the table and multiplying it by the $100 cash to be received in each period.

Amount Received × Present Value of Annuity of $1 = Product
$100 × 3.16987 = $316.99

	Amount Received	×	Present Value $1	=	Product
Year 1	$100	×	.90909	=	$ 90.91
Year 2	100	×	.82645	=	82.65
Year 3	100	×	.75131	=	75.13
Year 4	100	×	.68301	=	68.30
		Total			$316.99

Figure 16.5. Calculation of the present value of an ordinary annuity.

Use of present value tables allows one to further analyze financial information concerning potential capital acquisitions. It permits comparison of dollars spent today with future anticipated receipts restated in terms of present-day dollars.

Using information that was given earlier regarding the $500,000 equipment purchase with an expected 8-year life, analysis of relevant information concerning that purchase would contain the information shown in Figure 16.6.

Assuming cash flows will be discounted at 10%, this investment will generate a cash inflow in discounted dollars of $145,523, which should be interpreted to mean that in addition to yielding the business its 10% required return on investment, this equipment purchase is expected to generate an extra $145,523.

To determine the exact rate of return that was earned by the equipment, a reader need only divide $500,000 by the expected annual cash

Annual cash inflows generated by the machine $121,000

Factor for present value of annuity of $1
     For 8 periods at 10% × 5.3349
Present value of future cash inflows $645,523
    Less:
Cost of the equipment (500,000)*
     Net present value $145,523

*Brackets () are used to denote cash outflows.

Figure 16.6. Analysis of relevant information concerning a $500,000 equipment purchase.

inflows of $121,000. The quotient of 4.1212 can be taken back into the Present Value of an Ordinary Annuity of $1 table, across the 8 period line until a number approximating 4.1212 is found. The interest rate at the top of the column where the factor is found identifies the internal rate of return. In this problem, that factor would be located between 16% and 18%, informing the reader that this equipment generated a return that approximates 17%.

The discount rate selected directly affects equipment purchase decisions. This rate can be selected from several alternatives. One alternative is to use the entity's incremental borrowing rate (defined as that rate of interest that a lending institution would charge the hospital if it borrowed the equipment purchase price). In this way, entities can be assured that capital acquisitions will cover the costs associated with their purchase.

Entities can also use the rate of return that is associated with various investment opportunities that are currently available. A third alternative would be to use the profit rate that is currently being generated by the entity.

Ranking Equipment Requests

A positive net present value and a payback of five years or less are screening tools that hospitals use in their selection process. If requisitions exceed available resources, an entity needs to establish a method for prioritizing purchases. If there are no qualitative differences between proposed equipment purchases, a hospital should purchase those items that will yield the greatest return.

One measure of profitability is the internal rate of return that was described earlier. This method becomes more complex if cash inflows and outflows are different amounts and do not occur at regular time intervals.

Another method of ranking that could be used is one that ranks the quotients that are calculated by dividing an asset's net present value by the amount of its initial cash outlay. The higher the quotient, the higher the priority given to the equipment purchase. This method of ranking gives effect to the size of the original investment.

An entity may utilize its own methodology for ranking requests for new equipment. The methodology used for prioritizing should include only those equipment requests that satisfy all initial earnings criteria as exhibited by net present value calculations.

Qualitative Factors

Qualitative factors have been excluded from the aforementioned screening process. That is not to say that they can be completely ignored. A hospital has a mission of delivering quality patient care to its identified community. That mission cannot always be accomplished at a profit. Equipment purchase analysis should still be made even though an asset must be purchased for qualitative reasons and does not pass the initial screening. Information gathered may alert management to alternative methods of accomplishing the same goal. In any case, management should be aware of the cost that the hospital must bear as a result of decisions based upon qualitative factors.

SUMMARY

Fixed asset purchase decisions require more analysis than do operating decisions because invested amounts are greater and for longer time periods.

Two specific techniques that can be used to screen the various equipment requests are payback and net present value. Payback calculates how long it will take an institution to recoup its initial investment. Net present value computations are grounded upon the belief that there is a time value to money. This method calculates the present value of dollars that are expected to be generated or saved in future time periods. It reduces future receipts by the interest that is contained within future receipts. If present value of future receipts is greater than the equipment's purchase price, the purchase will be advantageous.

Limited institutional resources necessitate prioritizing new fixed asset requests. Screening tools help reduce the volume of eligible equipment requisition. In general, an institution should act upon those requests that will maximize profitability.

Qualitative issues play a role in purchase decisions. If a machine is purchased for qualitative reasons only, it is important to acknowledge the added cost associated with it.

QUESTIONS

1. How do capital acquisition decisions differ from operating decisions?

2. What is the payback method? What does it involve? What does its result tell the manager?
3. What is meant by discounting cash flows?
4. What is meant by the net present value method of analyzing capital acquisitions?
5. If there is a positive dollar amount identified as the net present value, what does it mean? What does a negative net present value amount mean?
6. What are the different rates that could be used in the discounting operation? Explain the rationale of each.

EXERCISES

1. The department has requested the purchase of a piece of equipment that will cost $10,000. It has an estimated useful life of five years and a residual value at the end of its life of $100. It will save supplies valued at $2,500 each year. The institution's cost of capital is 10%.

   Required:

   a) Calculate the payback period for the equipment.
   b) Calculate the net present value associated with the equipment.
   c) Should the institution purchase the equipment?
   d) Would your answer change if it were salary expense instead of supplies that were saved each year? What additional information, if any, would you need to make that decision?

2. The organization has received a request to purchase a new machine that costs $200,000. An old machine that cost $120,000 can be traded in for the new equipment. If that is done the manufacturer will reduce the invoice price by $2,000. The equipment has a useful life of 10 years. The department has generated the following cost and revenue information for the machine.

   New machine will perform 10,000 tests annually.

Fee charged per test	$6
Annual costs to operate:	
Required return on investment	10%
Salary of operator	$10,000
Supplies	5,500
Depreciation	20,000

Analyze the information given and decide whether the new machine should be purchased.

3. An alternative exists to purchasing the machine, which is to have the test sample taken in-house and sent to a neighboring laboratory. The costs involved in this alternative are given below.

Annual salary of sample gatherer	$6,000
Supplies	3,500
Fee charged by the laboratory	$4.00

Which alternative should the hospital select and why?

4. Equipment costing $40,000, with an expected life of 10 years, is requested for the new outpatient surgery suite. The manager of that department has prepared the following income projections. It is expected that the equipment will realize these projections each year of its life.

Income Statement for New Procedure		
Revenue		$20,000
Expenses:		
Salaries	$10,000	
Supplies	4,000	
Depreciation	4,000	(18,000)
Net Income		$ 2,000

The hospital requires an 8% rate of return on all of its investments. Calculate the following:

A. The payback period.
B. The new present value
C. Based upon your answers to A and B, would you recommend that this purchase be made?

    D. Is the internal rate of return higher or lower than 8%? Explain your answer.

    E. If Medicare utilization is 50% (the impact of Medicare patients has not been included in this analysis thus far), how will this affect the final answer and the purchase decision?

    F. What qualitative decisions will affect the decision to purchase the machine?

Glossary

ASSET   A resource that belongs to an entity and has future value beyond the present day.

BAD DEBTS   The balance of customer or patient accounts that are considered uncollectible because the patients are unwilling to pay the amount owed.

BALANCE SHEET   Financial statement that lists all of the assets, liabilities, and equity of an organization.

BUDGETING   The process of planning for the future and converting expected actions into expected revenues and expenses.

CAPITAL BUDGETING   The process of planning for major equipment and building acquisitions where costs are weighed against the benefits to be produced by the acquisition.

CASH FLOW STATEMENT   Financial statement that displays the changes in the cash balance according to their source. The sources considered are operating, investing, financing, and reclassifying.

CHARITY ALLOWANCE   The amounts owed by patients which are written off as uncollectible because the patients are unable to pay.

COINSURANCE   The amount that the patient is responsible for paying for each additional day's stay in the hospital.

CONSERVATISM   The viewpoint that accountants adopt that provides that all losses are included in the financial statements as soon as their occurrence is probable, but that gains are not recorded until they are a certainty.

CONSISTENCY   The general accounting principle that requires the same choice of generally accepted accounting principles from one time period to the next when there is a choice on the part of the entity.

This principle allows for changes, but requires full disclosure of the change and its effects when consistency is breached.

CONTRACTUAL ADJUSTMENT   The difference between the charged fee and the agreed-to price granted to specific insurance providers. Contractual adjustments are generally granted because they are legislated or because the contract provides for a high volume of services to be provided.

CORPORATION   A form of organization that involves legally registering the entity, thus making it a separate legal entity. Corporations have unlimited lifetimes.

COST   The generally accepted accounting principle that states that historical cost is the only objective supportable value for assets.

CURRENT ASSETS   Assets that are expected to be converted to cash or used up within one year or one operating cycle, whichever is greater.

CURRENT LIABILITIES   Any debt that is expected to be paid within one year or one operating cycle, whichever is greater. Current liabilities will be paid using current assets.

DEDUCTIBLE   The amount that is subtracted from the bill and designated as owed by the patient before insurance carriers are billed for any covered services.

DEPRECIATION   The allocation of the cost of a fixed asset to the time periods that it serves.

DIRECT LABOR   The labor involved in providing a service that involves direct patient contact.

DIRECT MATERIAL   The material or major supplies that become part of the end product or service.

DISCLOSURE   The generally accepted accounting principle that requires the inclusion of specific, relevant information in the body of the financial report. Where this information cannot be incorporated, it must be disclosed in the footnotes to the financial statements.

ENTITY   The accounting assumption that states that the business is separate and distinct from its owners.

EXPENSE   Any resource that is completely used up during the course of operations.

FIXED COST   Any cost that remains constant as the volume of services changes, thus causing a change in the unit cost of the service.

FOR-PROFIT CORPORATION   Corporation that is owned by shareholders who share the earnings of the entity in the form of dividends declared and paid.

GENERALLY ACCEPTED ACCOUNTING PRINCIPLES (GAAP)   Accounting rules that have been promulgated by the profession and accepted as the foundation of those statements by the users of financial statements.

GOING CONCERN   The accounting assumption that the entity is expected to continue operating as a business unless there is evidence to the contrary.

INCOME STATEMENT   Financial statement that lists the revenues, expenses, and resulting net income or loss of an entity. The end result is often termed excess of revenues over expenses for not-for-profit organizations.

JOB COSTING   A methodology for determining the cost of goods sold or services rendered by identifying the specific labor and material with the item produced.

LIABILITIES   Amounts owed to vendors and creditors.

LONG-TERM ASSETS   Assets that have a life of greater than one year.

MATCHING   The generally accepted accounting principle that states that all expenses must be included within the income statement if they were used to generate revenue during the period.

MATERIALITY   The generally accepted accounting principle that states that financial statements must be correct in all important aspects.

MEDICAID   Title XIX. Legislation that provides medical insurance to the nation's indigent population. Medicaid is supervised by state governments.

MEDICARE   Title XVIII. Legislation that provides medical insurance to the nation's elderly citizens, and selected individuals with kidney failure.

MIXED COST   A cost that contains an element of fixed cost and an element of variable cost.

NET PRESENT VALUE   The capital budgeting technique that provides a methodology for comparing two different cash flows with the purpose of determining whether an expenditure made today will generate sufficient future cash flows to pay for itself when the time value of money is considered a factor in the decision.

NOT-FOR-PROFIT CORPORATION   An entity that is organized as a separate legal entity, but whose purpose is to provide goods and services to a community. Any income generated by this entity is not available for distribution outside the entity.

OBJECTIVITY   Accounting assumption that requires verifiable, independently obtained information as support for accounting transactions before they can be recorded.

OVERHEAD   Any cost associated with operating a workplace that enables goods and services to be provided.

OWNERS' EQUITY   The owners' investment in the entity.

PARTNERSHIP   A form of organization that is evidenced by more than one owner. The entity has a life limited to that of any one of its partners and the partners share unlimited liability for all partnership debts.

PAYBACK   The capital budgeting technique that compares acquisition price with the expected future cash inflows to be generated by the equipment. The result tells the entity how long it will take for a piece of equipment to pay for itself, disregarding the time value of money concepts.

PERIODICITY The accounting assumption that allows the indefinite life of an entity to be divided into uniform periods of time so that financial statements can be prepared.

PROCESS COSTING The cost accounting methodology that spreads the costs of production (material, labor, and overhead) equitably over the units produced.

PROGRAM BUDGETING A budgeting process performed for a specific, limited time period that allows costs to be used in any way that generates the desired results.

REALIZATION The generally accepted accounting principle that states that revenue shall be recorded when the entity has substantially performed by either rendering a service or providing a good.

RELEVANT DATA Any information that changes between alternative courses of action.

RELEVANT RANGE That level of activity for which cost behavior patterns are expected to remain unchanged.

RELEVANT VALUE UNIT (RVU) The name given to the equivalent unit of production for a department that becomes the basis for defining the work performed and for spreading costs equitably over the different classes of units produced.

SOLE PROPRIETORSHIP An organization that is owned by one individual who accepts all risks and rewards associated with ownership.

STABLE DOLLAR The generally accepted accounting principle that specifies that all transactions be recorded using a common monetary unit that is not adjusted for changes in purchasing power.

STATEMENT OF EQUITY Financial statement that displays the change in the entity's equity account since the last financial report was prepared. Changes arise from income (increases), losses (decreases), and additional investment by owners.

VARIABLE COST   A cost that remains constant per unit of service. As the volume of service increases, total cost increases, and as the volume of service decreases, total cost decreases.

ZERO-BASED BUDGETING   Budgeting methodology that justifies every dollar of expense based upon expected activity and externally generated costs of providing services. A department has no base amount given to it and must construct the budget beginning with no dollars.

Index

Not-for-profit corporations, 26-27
Nursing differential, Medicare, 70
Nursing pools, 110

O

Objectivity assumption, generally accepted accounting principles (GAAP), 8
Omnibus Budget Reconciliation Act of 1981, 74
Operating budgets, 104
Opportunity costs, 161
Organizing, and budgeting, 98-99
Overhead analysis, 141-143
   fixed overhead, 143
   variable overhead, 142-143
Owners' equity account, 23
Owners' equity statement, 20-21
Ownership methods
   corporation, 25-27
   partnership, 24-25
   sole proprietorship, 23-24
Owners of business, use of financial information, 4-5

P

Partnership, nature of, 24-25
Patient charges, accounting treatment of, 35-36
Payback, 159-161
   example of, 160-161
Payroll, accounting treatment of, 37-38

Payroll withholding and payroll taxes, as liability, 19
Performance evaluation, and budgeting, 99-100
Periodicity assumption, generally accepted accounting principles (GAAP), 9
Planning, and budgeting, 98
Prepaid expenses, as asset, 18
Present value tables, 162-165
Preventive medicine, 77
Process costing, 137-139
   and relative value units, 137-139
Products, cost components, 133-135
Program budgeting, 105, 105-106
Property, as long-term asset, 18-19
Prospective payment system, 76
   excluded providers, 76
Provider Reimbursement Review Board, 71
Public Law 92-603, 70

R

Ranking equipment requests, 166
Realization principle, generally accepted accounting principles (GAAP), 11-12
Reasonable charges, 66-67
Regression analysis, mixed costs, 87-88
Relative value units, 89
   and process costing, 137-139
Replacement time, employee replacement, 110
Restricted donations, 41